How to Fight Arthritis & Win

How to Fight Arthritis & Win
Published by Agora Health Books
Alice Jacob, Managing Editor
Ken Danz, Copy Editor

ISBN 1-891434-12-8
Printed in the United States of America

AGORA HEALTH BOOKS
819 N. Charles St.
Baltimore, MD 21201
www.agorahealthbooks.com

HOW TO FIGHT ARTHRITIS & WIN

The *BEST* natural ways to successfully manage pain
and prevent the progression of arthritis

WILLIAM L. FISCHER

AGORA HEALTH BOOKS
BALTIMORE, MARYLAND

TABLE OF CONTENTS

FOREWARD i

INTRODUCTION iii

PREFACE v

CHAPTER 1
Understanding Osteoarthritis and
Rheumatoid Arthritis 1

CHAPTER 2
Your Arthritis Management Plan 27

CHAPTER 3
Eating for Joint Support and Pain Management 35

CHAPTER 4
Natural Relief With Nutritional
Supplements and Herbs 65

CHAPTER 5
Exercise—Make It Part of Your Life 107

CHAPTER 6
Bodywork and Topical Therapies 123

EPILOGUE 135

APPENDIX 1
Resources 137

APPENDIX 2
Bibliography 145

INDEX 148

FOREWORD

A man in his early 50s walked into his doctor's office and complained that his left knee was hurting. The doctor briefly examined the knee, added some notes to the man's file, and said, "Well, it looks like it might be arthritis. It's just a part of growing older." The patient sat there for a moment then replied, "But Doc, my right knee is just as old and it doesn't hurt".

One of the most unfortunate and biggest myths in our society is that we must accept arthritis as an inevitable part of aging. If this were the case, how could we explain the fact that many people don't contract arthritis and sail through to their 80s and 90s with nary a joint pain? What are their secrets to an arthritis-free life?

The truth is that suffering from arthritis need not be inevitable. In many cases, we can prevent this painful joint disease and live our lives without being burdened by it. In fact, with proper diet, proper exercise, and a little determination, you may never have to know just how painful this condition—which seems to be reaching epidemic proportions in the United States—can be.

That may sound like a bold statement. Once you have read this book, however, you will understand exactly why I say this. *How to Fight Arthritis & Win* can empower and give hope to those who suffer with this disease. It can give those who have not yet shown any signs of the condition a chance to prevent it. The fact is that with a tool like the book you hold in your hands you *can* fight arthritis and win.

The most wonderful aspect of this book is its emphasis on natural means and complementary medicine. Antiarthritic drugs are some of the most potent and potentially dangerous drugs a person can take. In many cases, they can cause a host of adverse side effects, some of which, in fact, are as painful as the condition itself. The remedies provided in this book, however, explain how to help your body rid itself of this joint disease and manage pain without succumbing to such strong medication.

How to Fight Arthritis & Win is an encouraging book that will help every person who reads it, whether he or she has arthritis, knows someone who has it, or is searching for ways to prevent the appearance of it or its progression.

I am delighted that a book of this sort has finally been written. With its simple, easy-to-read presentation and its actionable and easy to implement suggestions, it is long overdue.

Tom McCabe, RPIH

INTRODUCTION

Your fingers ache, your back hurts, it takes awhile for you to get moving in the morning, and aches and pains during the night are preventing you from getting a good night's rest. This is what a mild case of arthritis feels like. Some people have arthritis so severe, however, that their fingers are disfigured and are practically useless. It is difficult for them to get up and move around, no matter the time of day, because their bones and joints hurt so bad and are so stiff. This is arthritis at its worst.

The word "arthritis" encompasses literally hundreds of different ailments, including gout, bursitis, carpal tunnel syndrome, and tendinitis. Explained in the simplest of terms, it is a degenerative process of the joints that is often accompanied by inflammation and pain.

The two most common forms of arthritis are osteoarthritis and rheumatoid arthritis. We will discuss these in more detail in the first chapter. Although much progress has been made in terms of diagnosis and the identification of at least some risk factors, these two conditions still remain largely a mystery to the medical community. No one is quite sure what causes them.

And the diseases remain a mystery to those who suffer from them as well. For example, osteoarthritis can be merely a nuisance for some people for many years— but in others it can rapidly progress into a crippling condition. Rheumatoid arthritis is equally puzzling.

Flareups come and go, and it often follows an erratic course, remaining relatively minor for several years and then suddenly growing extremely worse, for no explainable reason.

These are only two forms of this common problem. However, they can manifest themselves in a variety of ways. Some of the ailments described in this book may seem to have little in common, while others are closely related in terms of cause and in the course of their development. This book was written not only to provide you with a better understanding of the major forms of arthritis, but also as a tool to help you take control over your health and life once again.

PREFACE

Taking the time and making the effort to fight arthritis and reverse its toll on your life is worth every second it takes. After all, why should you stop doing the things you love if you don't have to? Not only that, but arthritis tends to be a progressive disease. Even if you think the discomfort is tolerable now, for how long will it be tolerable? I encourage you, with this book as your guide, to fully embrace the idea that you can and will claim your life back from arthritis and not be its victim.

Fighting arthritis can make all the difference. Consider Rose and Mary, for example, two longtime friends. Twenty years ago, Mary was turning 50 when her osteoarthritis took a turn for the worse. Accepting her fate and helplessness, she agreed to have her first hip replacement. Rose, who is 10 years older than Mary, was diagnosed with osteoarthritis at about the same time. But Rose, witnessing her friend's suffering, said to herself, "Not if I can help it!" She added supplements to her diet, lost some weight, and started a steady regimen of dance classes for exercise. Though she succeeded at keeping arthritis at bay, Rose unfortunately failed to convince Mary that there were many things she could do to make the situation better. Today, 20 years later, Mary has endured successive surgeries, pain, and powerful painkillers. Rose, on the other hand, is still dancing.

This book brings you the best of natural medicine from across the world, as well as other time-tested remedies that will help you overcome arthritis. It covers the treatment and prevention of arthritis in two ways: (a) reducing pain and supporting joints from the "inside out," through healthful eating and the use of, nutritional supplements and herbal remedies and (b) from the "outside in," through exercise, bodywork, and topical formulas.

It is exciting to start any journey—and you have begun the greatest journey of all, that of taking control of your health.

Good luck and good health!

William L. Fischer

• CHAPTER 1 •

Understanding Osteoarthritis and Rheumatoid Arthritis

Over 10 years ago, a popular weekly news magazine called arthritis "the nation's primary crippler." More than a decade later, despite millions spent on research and mountains of medicine, the news is the same—arthritis is *still* the nation's primary crippler.

Indeed, the statistics make one's head spin. The Arthritis Foundation estimates that over 21 million Americans suffer from osteoarthritis alone. When you add rheumatoid arthritis to the mix, along with the many other joint conditions, the number of patients doubles. One in three families, amounting to one-third of the nation's households, is touched in some way by the condition. And the problem is not letting up. More than a million new cases are diagnosed every year.

Additionally, arthritis costs the nation billions of dollars each year in lost workdays, medication, surgery, and home-nursing services. A medical disease of such magnitude needs our understanding. What is it? What causes it? And perhaps the most important question of all: Can we prevent it or alleviate it?

This chapter deals with understanding the two most common types of arthritis: *osteoarthritis* and *rheumatoid arthritis*. According to the Arthritis Foundation, there are more than 100 different types of arthritis or arthritis-related conditions. In this chapter, you will learn about several of the more common forms affecting the body's joints and some surprising information about what may be causing your pain or making it worse.

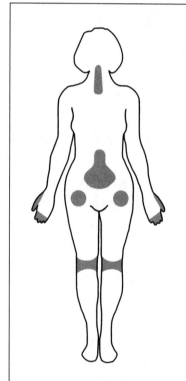

Areas of the Body Osteoarthritis Affects

Osteoarthritis most often occurs at the ends of the fingers, thumbs, neck, lower back, knees, and hips.

Illustration courtesy of the National Institute of Arthritis and Musculoskeletal and Skin Diseases (NIAMS)

Osteoarthritis (OA)

Osteoarthritis—the most common form of this widespread medical problem—is characterized by pain and stiffness in the joints. In most people, it is limited to only one or two parts of the body (usually one or two of the following: fingers, knees, hips, lower back, or neck).

The disease usually hits a person around the age of 50, but X-rays reveal that the deterioration may begin as early as 20 years of age in some individuals. Unfortunately, it's fairly common. According to the National Institute of Arthritis and Musculoskeletal and Skin Diseases (NIAMS), nine out of 100 people in their 30s develop OA in their knees or hips. By the age of 40, about nine out of 10 people experience some arthritic changes in their weight-bearing joints, and after age 55, virtually everyone will experience some joint pain and stiffness—the hallmarks of osteoarthritis. NIAMS has found that the occurrence of arthritis rises twofold to tenfold from age 30 to age 65.

Women seem to be more prone to develop it in their fingers first, while men tend to get it in their hips. Osteoarthritis usually strikes both sides of the body. If you feel pain in your right knee, you can soon expect the left knee to begin hurting as well. In general, the joint on the dominant side of the body is affected first.

Types of Osteoarthritis

There are two basic types of osteoarthritis—primary and secondary. The primary variety is the kind that "just happens" for no apparent reason. You wake up one morning with a stiff, sore shoulder, but you don't know why. And the stiffness and pain stay with you. This is the type of arthritis people are referring to when they talk about "wear and tear" on the body. It feels as if the joints are just wearing out. This common, simple explanation, though, does not address the question of why some people acquire osteoarthritis and others do not.

By contrast, secondary osteoarthritis has a definite cause. It could develop because of a fracture or similar injury to the bones and joints early in life; an infection in the joint; overuse of drugs injected into the joint; tissue damage caused by disease, such as diabetes; or deposits of calcium in the cartilage.

Understanding Osteoarthritis

To understand osteoarthritis, you need to know how the joints work.

Bones meet inside a joint capsule. The ends of the bones are lubricated and cushioned so they can slide past each other to assume either flexed or straightened positions. The capsule itself is made of tough fibrous tissue. Muscles taper down to become *tendons* and attach to the bone at the joint. The ends of bones, located inside this joint capsule, are protected and lubricated by the *synovial membrane*.

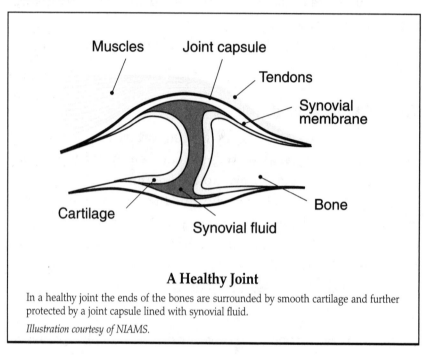

Muscles   Joint capsule   Tendons   Synovial membrane   Cartilage   Bone   Synovial fluid

A Healthy Joint

In a healthy joint the ends of the bones are surrounded by smooth cartilage and further protected by a joint capsule lined with synovial fluid.

Illustration courtesy of NIAMS.

The end of the bone is covered by a smooth layer of cartilage that allows for ease of movement. Osteoarthritis causes this very important cartilage to flake and wear away.

In certain joints of the body, small pouches filled with a gummy fluid supply extra lubrication for the body's tissues. These are called *bursae*. When the bursae become inflamed, the condition is known as *bursitis*. Bursitis most often occurs in the shoulder but can also affect the knee, elbow, Achilles tendon, foot, and other areas.

Looking at the structure in more detail, we find that at the heart of the joint are two bones that meet and move. The tip of each bone is covered with a smooth layer of cartilage that creates a smooth frictionless surface, allowing the bones to slide easily and absorb shock. It is this cartilage that is affected in osteoarthritis. In the beginning stages of the condition, the swollen cartilage begins to flake. Over time, deep vertical cracks appear. The cartilage cells attempt to repair this damage by accumulating around the cracks, but the cells are unsuccessful. In fact, instead of helping the joint, this attempt by the body to repair itself puts it under considerable strain.

In a further attempt to protect itself, the body then lays down extra calcium at the outer ends of the bone—where the tendons and ligaments are attached. Consequently, small bony spurs, called *osteophytes*, form inside the joints. They are most visible as bony knobs (*Heberden's nodes*) at the end of the finger joints.

Making matters worse, a jolt or twist may occasionally break off an osteophyte allowing it to move about inside the joint space. It is possible for an unattached osteophyte to get caught between the two bones as they move, causing an extremely painful condition.

During this degenerative process, the synovial membrane covering the joint is affected as well. The membrane's blood vessels narrow, thus reducing the blood flow. As the joint is used, the friction creates heat. The flow of blood is not adequate to dissipate the increasing heat. Moreover, the membrane stiffens when the joint is at rest. This condition, commonly referred to as "gelling," makes the joint difficult to move.

Symptoms of Osteoarthritis

Osteoarthritis, a degenerative disease, appears gradually in the body, usually affecting only a few joints in its initial stages. Early symptoms include a dull pain and stiffness in one or several joints. This condition is usually worse in the morning and gradually eases as the day progresses. After a relatively short period of time, however, the person will begin to notice that the pain recurs throughout the day and then, for no discernible reason, disappears. Moderate activity or stretching can usually ease the aches, but vigorous exercise or repetitive activity often increases the pain. For example, people who work on computers all day may complain about aches in their fingers and hands in the course of a long session at the keyboard. However, even when away from the computer, they may experience difficulty using their hands, such as when trying to button their coats or open jars.

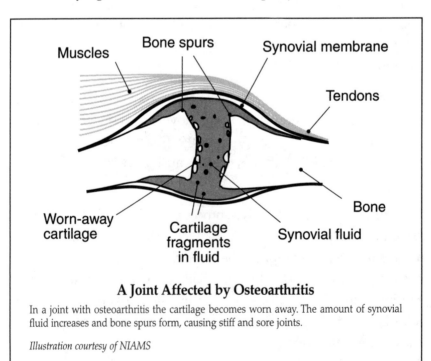

A Joint Affected by Osteoarthritis

In a joint with osteoarthritis the cartilage becomes worn away. The amount of synovial fluid increases and bone spurs form, causing stiff and sore joints.

Illustration courtesy of NIAMS

As the disease progresses, the pain lasts for longer periods of time. Activities that the person was once able to perform easily now involve much pain. In some instances, the person cannot do them at all. In addition, tenderness may exist and swelling may be present—as well as a redness and warmth around the affected joints.

In advanced cases of osteoarthritis, the joint may actually make a crepitant (popping or crunching) sound when it is moved. The range of motion becomes limited, and eventually certain joints may become deformed. Hands affected by this condition may become twisted due to the deviations of the small joints.

When the neck is affected by osteoarthritis, the disc spaces

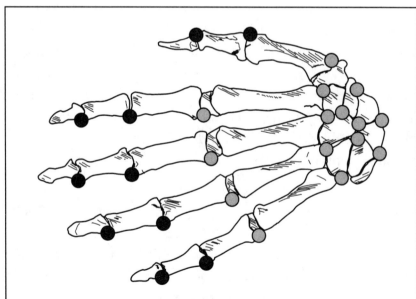

Arthritis in the Hand and Wrist

Osteoarthritis, denoted by the black circles, settles into the outermost joints of the hand. Rheumatoid arthritis, denoted by the light grey circles, by contrast, affects the lower joints of the hand and wrist.

Illustration courtesy of NIAMS

between the vertebrae are compressed due to a degenerative condition called *cervical spondylosis.* Among the indications of this process may be a pain that shoots from the back of the neck to the head or to the top of the shoulders. Pain may radiate to the hand. There may even be muscle weakness in the arm. Bony spurs that compress the nerves cause this weakness. In very rare cases, these spurs may compress vessels carrying blood to the brain, prompting neurological problems, and possibly even lead to a stroke.

Rheumatoid Arthritis

Rheumatoid arthritis differs greatly from osteoarthritis. Instead of affecting only one joint or the back, rheumatoid arthritis affects the entire body. For this reason, it is called a *systemic illness.*

Inflammation is a major factor in this type of arthritis. Not only do the joints become inflamed, but in many cases so do the eyes, lungs, heart, muscles, and even the nerves. The inflammation begins in the synovial membrane, which lines the joints. The membrane thickens and invades first the cartilage and eventually the bone. This process may damage the joints. Most commonly, the wrists, elbows, shoulders, knees, and hands are affected: more specifically, the small joints of the hands and knees are involved.

A person with rheumatoid arthritis endures the pain of hot, swollen joints. But accompanying this is a series of flulike symptoms—chills, fever, loss of appetite, loss of weight, fatigue, and a general malaise. Although the symptoms usually appear gradually, the onset is sudden in about 10 percent of the cases. In some people, it can develop as quickly as overnight.

About 40 percent of all rheumatoid-arthritis sufferers are affected in the spine. It usually hurts when a patient moves his or her head. For some people, the pain is so severe that it even radiates to the forehead. Others cannot tilt their heads backward because of the pain and the accompanying tingling sensation in the arms.

In addition to experiencing pain and malaise, many people develop disfiguring nodules under the skin. Ranging in size from a small pea to a pearl onion, these nodules signal the inflammation of a blood vessel. Most often, they appear just below the elbow or over some other bony prominence. In some instances, the nodules may form over a bursa or tendon.

Rheumatoid arthritis is a potentially lethal disease, but fortunately it seldom develops to such a serious state. About 20 percent

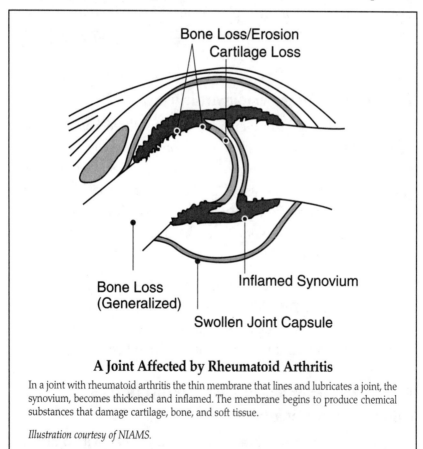

A Joint Affected by Rheumatoid Arthritis

In a joint with rheumatoid arthritis the thin membrane that lines and lubricates a joint, the synovium, becomes thickened and inflamed. The membrane begins to produce chemical substances that damage cartilage, bone, and soft tissue.

Illustration courtesy of NIAMS.

of those who develop the disease recover from it with no adverse side effects. Another 20 percent suffer permanent joint damage. The majority of those who get rheumatoid arthritis will be bothered by occasional flareups and periodic joint pain.

The rheumatoid version of arthritis, unlike osteoarthritis, is most often a disease of the young, normally affecting those between the ages of 25 and 50. However, it can strike older people as well.

About 75 percent of those affected are women. Why women are more frequently the victims is a mystery. But medical experts suspect that hormones may play a part. Rheumatoid arthritis will frequently ease and in some instances disappear during pregnancy only to recur after the baby is born.

The Patterns of Rheumatoid Arthritis

Rheumatoid arthritis generally follows three basic patterns: *monocyclic, polycyclic, and chronic.* In the monocyclic pattern, the arthritis lasts for several months at a time and then goes away. The polycyclic version consists of several shorter attacks. Between these attacks, the person will feel fine. With chronic rheumatoid arthritis, the most prevalent type, the patient feels some type of discomfort most of the time.

In all three of these patterns, the disease becomes less aggressive as the years pass. You feel less tired and less stiff the longer you have the arthritis. As time passes, the inflammation of the synovial membrane lessens and no new joints are involved.

Possible Causes of Rheumatoid Arthritis (RA) and Other Arthritic Conditions

Doctors are not sure exactly what causes rheumatoid arthritis and other rheumatic and arthritic conditions, but they do have several theories. Among these theories, three have garnered the most attention:

(1) It is caused by a malfunction in the immune system, which causes it to attack the body.

(2) It is caused by viruses.

(3) It is caused by the aggravation of stress upon the body.

Immune Malfunction

The first theory, involving a dysfunction in the immune system, is the one most widely held by the medical community.

A properly functioning immune system produces cells that defend the body against things that are foreign to it—such as viruses and germs. It does this either through innate immunity, in which the body instantly recognizes the foreign invader and kills it, or through *adaptive immunity*. The latter form occurs when the body is taught to recognize a virus through the process of vaccination.

But if the cells malfunction, they can attack normal healthy parts of the body. These cells are filled with a digestive enzyme that surrounds and engulfs what your system perceives to be a foreign invader. When that happens, you have an *autoimmune disease*. In other words, your body's immune system mistakes its own tissues to be pathogens or foreign invaders and attacks itself.

The reason the body begins to attack itself in certain people is not clear yet. However, researchers have discovered the existence of a gene called HLA-DR4 that is involved with the immune system's ability to recognize foreign substances. This gene, whether normal or defective, may be implicated in the development of rheumatoid arthritis. Research on the genetic causes of RA continues.

The Virus Theory

Another popular theory as to the cause of the immune malfunction seen in RA is the virus theory. Scientists speculate that a virus can settle into a joint and cause inflammation. If it penetrates into tissue cells, the body's defenses may not be able to tell the difference between the virus and the person's own tissue.

Although the virus theory is generally associated with RA, it is increasingly recognized that viruses and some bacteria may also exacerbate osteoarthritis and other arthritis-type conditions regardless of whether or not they initially cause the arthritis.

Mycoplasmas: Tiny Microorganisms That Could Be Causing Your Arthritis

One genus of bacteria that researchers have been studying as a possible trigger for the symptoms of arthritis is mycoplasma. In 2001, the Health Sciences Institute (see page 138 for more information about this institution) published a revealing report on mycoplasma and its implication in arthritis. Mycoplasmas are tiny microorganisms. They are bacteria commonly found in the saliva and mucous membranes of the mouth or nose, and they were once dismissed as relatively harmless organisms. However, it's been discovered that mycoplasmas may also penetrate into blood cells—where they are far from harmless. It's theorized that painful joints may actually be the result of a systemic infection caused by this tiny microorganism.

Researchers have made the surprising discovery that mycoplasmal infections occur in approximately half of the patients with certain chronic diseases—including arthritis.

It's relatively simple to test for the presence of mycoplasmas on mucosal surfaces like the mouth. Once they get inside cells, however, conventional antibody tests are usually useless, and they are extremely difficult to culture.

Fortunately, a newly developed and specialized test, called a forensic PCR-DNA, is able to detect fragments of mycoplasmas inside the white blood cells. The white blood cells scavenge those pieces as they clean up debris in the tissues and blood. If the DNA of a mycoplasma is found in your white blood cells, an active infection exists. (**Note:** Labs that conduct PCR-DNA testing for mycoplasma are listed in Appendix I.)

So what can you do if you test positive for a mycoplasmal infection? The conventional treatment for such an infection is strong antibiotic therapy.

Antibiotics are effective, but the course of treatment may last many months. If you choose the antibiotic approach, expect a period of die-off symptoms lasting as long as two months. As the bacteria are killed, toxins flood the bloodstream as they are discarded and symptoms become temporarily worse.

Darryl See, M.D., has for several years now been treating patients with such infections at the Center for Special Immunology and also at the Chronic Fatigue Syndrome and Fibromyalgia Clinic at UC Irvine, which he co-directs.

In his own practice, Dr. See has observed that patients' PCR-DNA tests can turn from positive to negative when they are treated with colloidal silver. However, he stresses that not all colloidal-silver products are the same. The colloidal silver used by Dr. See contains three to five parts silver per million, and the particles of silver are dissolved to the tiny molecular size of 2 to 5 nanometers. It appears that the smaller size may be more effective against mycoplasmas than are the more common colloidal silvers with particles ranging from 50 to 100 ppm (parts per million). And since less silver is consumed on a daily basis, toxicity is rare.

A number of experts recommend selenium and oxygen supplements to combat a mycoplasmal infection. A dose of 200 to 400 micrograms of selenium as a dietary supplement has been shown to arrest the growth of the invaders. Also, because mycoplasmas

> **T I P**
>
> If you have been diagnosed with rheumatoid arthritis that appears to be worsening, be sure to consult with your doctor. Although a mild problem for most people, rheumatoid arthritis can escalate into a chronic condition.

prefer an environment low in oxygen, providing extra oxygen through magnesium-peroxide supplements may inhibit their growth.

The research on the mycoplasma/arthritis connection has just begun—but it's already clear that these mysterious creatures probably play an important role in arthritis. If mycoplasmas are attacking your joints, eliminating them from your system may help you beat arthritis for good.

Stress and the Toll It Takes on Health

Doctors who research the causes of rheumatoid arthritis are learning that, in addition to its possibly being caused by an injury to a joint, an infection, or a weakened physical state, the disease may be caused by, or at least aggravated by, stress. It is recognized that emotional disturbances and stressful events can precipitate a breakdown in health, be it the onset of migraines, stomach disorders, or other health conditions. The same appears to be true of rheumatoid arthritis. Chronic stress or a traumatic event, and how the individual responds to it, may be an underlying cause of RA attacks.

In one study, doctors discovered that stress precipitated an attack in almost 50 percent of the 293 people involved. In another project, doctors instructed rheumatoid-arthritis sufferers to keep "life charts," records of their attacks as well as stressful events. In 62 percent of the cases, a relationship between stress and RA attacks was found.

If stress is indeed contributing to your RA attacks, you may be able to lessen the severity and perhaps even the frequency of the attacks by learning to better handle the stressful situations in your life. Doctors emphasize that a stressful event is not limited to unpleasant occurrences. Joyous moments, such as the marriage of a child and beginning that new job you always dreamed of, can be just as difficult on the nerves.

If you suspect that your rheumatoid-arthritis episodes are either caused or aggravated by stress, keep your own "life chart." It is easy to do. Get a calendar or notebook large enough to make notations on specific days. Keep track of your arthritis flareups as well as any other notable events from those days. There is no need to make a notation for every day (if this is too time consuming), just for those days when a bout of arthritis occurs.

On the next page is an example of what tracking arthritis flareups in your daily calendar might look like:

What to Do About Stress

If you find a correlation between your arthritis and the stressful situations in your life, you need to find ways to either eliminate the sources of stress or learn how to manage it more effectively.

Not all stress can be alleviated easily. Life, as we all know, is

WEEKLY PLANNER

MONDAY: I FINISHED MY ANNUAL REPORT.

THE STAFF MEETING DID NOT GO WELL.

I FELT PAIN IN MY LEFT SHOULDER AND MY LOWER BACK.

I HAD A DINNER MEETING WITH JONES & COMPANY

TUESDAY: IT WAS TIME TO SIGN A NEW CONTRACT. MY BACK AND SHOULDER PAIN WAS WORSE THIS MORNING

I GOT THE CONTRACT WITH JONES & COMPANY

WEDNESDAY: IT WAS FAMILY NIGHT

I DID NOT NOTICE ANY PAIN WHEN I WOKE UP

THURSDAY: TODAY WAS OUR COMPANY PICNIC

I FELT NO PAIN THIS MORNING

FRIDAY: IT WAS RAINING VERY HARD AND I HAD TO DRIVE TO MEET NEW CLIENT.

MY SHOULDER PAIN WAS VERY BAD THIS MORNING.

SATURDAY: I VISITED MY IN-LAWS IN THE MORNING AND CUT THE LAWN IN THE AFTERNOON.

I WENT OUT TO DINNER WITH JOAN AND PAUL AND HIRED A SITTER FOR THE KIDS.

EXPERIENCED PAIN IN SHOULDER AND BACK IN MORNING BUT IT WENT AWAY AS DAY WENT ON. NONE AT BEDTIME.

full of various kinds of stress. While it may require discipline and determination on your part, the best approach is to learn to manage your reactions to stress rather than trying to control the factors that cause it. There are lots of resources available to help you do just that. Choose something that fits well into your schedule and fits comfortably into your lifestyle. You can try a relaxation or yoga class, a tension-taming book, or even a CD of guided relaxation. Also, in Chapter 5 and Chapter 6 I discuss a number of ways to promote relaxation and reduce stress.

Routines Can Be Helpful

Cultivate a routine. This may help you cope better with the stresses of your day and, in turn, help to reduce the severity and frequency of your rheumatoid-arthritis attacks.

While routines have a bad reputation as being boring and dull, they can actually be a blessing for an arthritis sufferer. A routine gives a person the feeling of being in control of his life. If, for example, the first thing you do every morning is make the bed, that act helps to establish a sense of order in your life.

Be sure, in creating your routine, to factor in at least 30 minutes each day to do nothing. Pick a time during the day that will be the easiest time for you to stick to your "do-nothing" commitment. You may want to time it to coincide with your favorite television show; that way, you have a reason to stop whatever it is you are doing.

This period of time should require little, if any, physical or mental energy. It should be a time when you can just lie on the couch and relax. Your body and your mind deserve this peaceful 30-minute respite. And you will be surprised at your ambition, enthusiasm, and energy once you give yourself permission to include this relaxing break into your schedule.

Other Related Diseases

Juvenile Rheumatoid Arthritis

About 300,000 children are affected by juvenile rheumatoid arthritis, according to one recent estimate by the Arthritis Foundation. The cause of this disease is unknown, and, in fact, the three types now recognized may really be three different diseases.

About half of the children affected have the polyarticular variety, in which only a single joint is affected. Another one-third of those with juvenile arthritis have several joints involved (usually including the knees). The multiple-joint variety usually disappears on its own by the time the child has reached his teens. The remaining one-sixth of those affected have Still's Disease. With this type of rheumatoid arthritis, the child may suddenly become seriously ill— running a high temperature accompanied by a rash and swelling of the lymph nodes. An accurate diagnosis may be difficult, because the joints may appear to be unaffected.

Systemic Lupus Erythematosus

Very little is known about the cause of this condition, and for that reason medical science has yet to develop a cure for systemic lupus erythematosus.

In this disease, a process occurs whereby the body produces antibodies that end up attacking its own tissues. This process strikes not only the joints and the skin but also blood vessels, the lining of the heart, the lungs, and other internal organs. The destruction of tissue often results.

Lupus is characterized by a unique, butterfly-shaped rash that appears on a person's nose and cheeks. This is often one of the earliest signs of the disease. Joint pain is reported by more than 90 percent of those affected with this condition. Arthritic deformities, however, rarely occur.

Women develop this ailment more often than men. For every man who acquires this condition, eight or nine women do. While it is not considered a rare disease, systemic lupus erythematosus affects only about one in more than 1,000 persons.

Doctors diagnose the presence of lupus by use of a blood test that reveals the presence of abnormal antibodies, a sign that the body is attacking itself.

Psoriatic Arthritis

Psoriatic arthritis was not recognized as a medical condition until the late 1920s. Very similar to rheumatoid arthritis, it is a condition in which several joints become inflamed. The inflammation is often accompanied by pain, redness, swelling, and warmth.

Most commonly, the smaller joints of the fingers and toes are affected. The nails may become pitted with depressions or ridges and sometimes become detached. Other areas of the skin may become affected by an inflammatory skin condition called psoriasis that is characterized by redness, itching, and thick dry silvery gray scales on the skin. The fingers and toes often show severe swelling. Although psoriatic arthritis is considered relatively rare, approximately one in 20 individuals with psoriasis will go on to develop arthritis.

In the typical case of psoriatic arthritis, the person will develop psoriasis first. It takes another 10 or 12 years for the joints to become painful. According to a Mayo clinic study those with the most severe skin problems are most likely to acquire this form of arthritis. Once the disease is established, the skin and joint symptoms will emerge and recede together.

Ankylosing Spondylitis

The name may not be familiar, but the condition known as ankylosing spondylitis has been documented since the third century B.C. Also known as Marie Strumpell disease, named after the 19th century scientist who was the first person to **fully** describe the condition, this ailment is also referred to as "poker spine."

In extreme cases of ankylosing spondylitis, bone can form between the vertebrae of the spine and eventually fuse the spine, skull, ribs, and hips into a long bone, which cannot be bent. The condition seldom gets that severe, however. Most commonly, pain and stiffness occur in the lower back and hip. The onset of the symptoms is quite gradual, and they can become worse at night or after periods of inactivity. As the condition slowly develops, the pain increases and the back may remain stiff for several days. Then, unexplainably, the symptoms disappear. This pattern of symptoms and remissions will then repeat periodically.

The disease eventually will travel up the spine. In about one-third of the cases, joints in the arms or legs will become inflamed. Other symptoms can include a loss of appetite with corresponding weight loss and an occasional low-grade fever.

As the condition progresses, it may also affect the *sacroiliac,* the joint of the lower back where the small triangular bone located just above the buttocks meets the hipbone. Fusing may also develop in the joints where the ribs meet the backbone.

As these joints become inflamed, fibrous tissue grows from the synovial membrane and into the cartilage lining of the joint. The joint space will, over time, become filled with this material. At the same time, the bones near the joint also become inflamed and harden. Eventually, the joint space is transformed into solid bone. The vertebrae and discs of the spine are also fused together.

In its initial stages, ankylosing spondylitis is often very painful. After the fusing has taken place, however, the pain normally disappears and only the stiffness remains. If the ribs and spine are fused, deep breathing can be difficult because chest expansion is limited. In severe cases, the heart's aortic valve may not function properly and cavities may develop in the lungs. In the vast majority of cases, the condition does not develop that far: Most people with the problem live active, full lives.

Most people who suffer from ankylosing spondylitis are young men, some as young as 15 years of age. It may remain undiagnosed, however, until the man reaches his late 30s or early 40s. It is rare for this condition to affect women, and, when it does, the ailment rarely progresses past a very mild case.

Ankylosing spondylitis appears to be a hereditary disease. In more than 50 percent of the cases, there is a family history of the disorder.

Gout

Gout was once called the disease of kings, referring to its association with an overindulgent diet too rich in fatty meats, expensive seafood, and alcohol. Advances in research and medicine have made this disease highly treatable. Approximately 275 of every 100,000 people suffer from this painful condition every year.

Gout is an arthritic condition that develops when too much uric acid builds up in the body. The uric acid crystallizes and deposits in joints, causing inflammation and pain. Gout can develop very quickly with a severe painful attack that includes redness, swelling, warmth, and tenderness in a joint. Initially it affects only one joint at a time, typically the big toe. An untreated attack of gout will often subside after a week or two, and periods between attacks can last months or even years. Eventually, the attacks become more frequent and severe and can spread to more joints.

Uric acid is a normal byproduct of the process the body goes through to break down waste products called purines. An excess of uric acid in the body could be caused either by a failure on the part of the kidneys to eliminate the acid efficiently or by an intake of foods that are high in purine, including certain meats, seafood, dried peas, and beans. Other dietary factors that can lead to gout are crash diets and the drinking of too much alcohol. An attack of gout also may appear after a severe illness, following surgery, or after one experiences a joint injury. Gout is often associated with obesity, hypertension, high cholesterol, and diabetes. The tendency toward gout may be inherited in some people.

While everyone is at risk for developing gout, men over 40 are hit with it most often. Women who develop gout tend to do so more often after menopause.

Fibromyalgia

Fibromyalgia is a somewhat mysterious and often misunderstood arthritis-related condition. While it is not considered to be an actual form of arthritis, it is strongly associated with it and is classified as a soft-tissue rheumatic condition. The syndrome presents itself not with an inflammation but rather with pain and stiffness in the joints, muscles, and bones. It is estimated that about 2 percent of the U.S. population suffers from the condition.

In the past, the condition was so misunderstood that sufferers were sometimes told that the pain was all in their heads and not real. However, medical studies proved the existence of the condition, and finally, in 1990, the American College of Rheumatology presented guidelines for diagnosing it. A doctor can make the diagnosis if he or she finds that you have had a history of widespread pain for at least a three-month period of time and pain in at least 11 of 18 specific tender points on the body.

Arthritis Associated With Inflammatory Bowel Diseases

Arthritis can occur as a complication of some forms of bowel disease, most often ulcerative colitis and regional enteritis; the latter is a term that includes such conditions as Crohn's disease, granulomatous colitis, and other forms of colitis.

Persons suffering with any of these conditions are more likely to acquire ankylosing spondylitis (see the previous section for information on this disorder) or peripheral arthritis, an arthritic condition affecting the joints in the limbs or the spine.

Approximately 15 percent of all ulcerative-colitis sufferers develop peripheral arthritis, usually in the knees and ankles. Attacks last about four to eight weeks but are infrequent. Similarly, ankylosing spondylitis is a hundred times more common in people with colitis than in the general public. The relationship between these two conditions is not clear.

Carpal Tunnel Syndrome

An inflammation of the tube through which the tendons pass is called *tenosynovitis* and is usually the result of trauma. One of the most commonly diagnosed types of tenosynovitis is *carpal tunnel syndrome.*

With this specific problem, which affects mostly middle-aged women, pain is felt with wrist movement, usually shooting down the fingers and up the forearm. The three middle fingers of the affected area often feel tingly and numb.

The size of the tunnel, or tube, which the nerve passes through is reduced due to the thickening of the tendon sheaths and arthritic changes of the wrist. The nerve, which is softer than the tendons, is subjected to considerable pressure and corresponding discomfort.

If pressure upon the nerve has been present for a considerable time, the person affected with carpal tunnel syndrome will notice a feeling of clumsiness when he attempts very fine movements. The person may drop dishes, for example. Pain is usually worse at night. The individual may be awakened by discomfort in the hand, which only exercise will alleviate.

Now that you have a clearer picture of some of the most common forms of arthritis and arthritis-related conditions, the following chapters will provide you with winning tools and techniques for fighting it.

• CHAPTER 2 •

Your Arthritis Management Plan

For most people, getting treated for arthritis consists of going to the doctor and taking pills, taking more pills to ease the uncomfortable side effects of the first pills, and then, later on, submitting to painful invasive surgery.

But what if this unhappy cycle could be reversed so that an arthritis sufferer could see himself or herself on a trajectory back to well-being?

After all...

Arthritis is a disease with symptoms that can be affected either *positively or negatively* by almost every aspect of your lifestyle— what you eat and drink, how you exercise (or if you don't), how you respond to stress, and your attitude.

Your best bet for fighting arthritis is to create and follow a personalized arthritis-management plan that helps you take back your life. In other words, you need to manage your arthritis so it doesn't manage you. It's not as hard as you might think and this book will help you do it. In fact, what's much harder is suffering from arthritis and <u>not</u> doing anything about it. Taking action is a step in the right direction.

Natural Healing – Helping the Whole Body, Not Just a Body Part

There was a popular song some years ago that went something like this: "The hand bone's connected to the wrist bone, the wrist bone's connected to the arm bone, the arm bone's connected to the shoulder bone…" and so on until it covered the entire body. Well, that old song pretty much sums up the concept behind holistic and natural healing—all parts of the body are connected to one another. When something happens to any one part of the body, the whole body is affected for better or for worse.

The big bonus of a natural-healing arthritis plan is that the benefits don't stop at alleviating arthritis and joint pain. Many of the arthritis-fighting methods provided here will also support and promote good health for your heart, your digestion, your circulation, and your overall well-being.

A Prescription for Disaster?

Taking strong pharmaceutical medicines for arthritis and joint pain may alleviate symptoms in the short term, but the long-term toll on your health and life can be as devastating as the arthritis they were meant to relieve in the first place.

Recent headlines have been particularly disturbing. The Aug. 22, 2001, issue of the *Journal of the American Medical Association (JAMA)* released an analysis of research involving Cox-2 inhibitors (such as Vioxx and Celebrex). The conclusion drawn was that patients taking these medicines may be at an increased risk for heart disease (up to a 50 percent or 60 percent greater risk according to two different studies). Cox-2 inhibitors have been heavily promoted as a "safer" class of medication for arthritis patients because during testing they purportedly took less of a toll on the digestive track. These tests, of course, failed to take fully into account some of the other health problems the drugs may contribute to. In response to the revelation that the Cox-2 inhibitors may be negatively affecting heart health, some doctors are suggesting that patients taking these medicines also take aspirin to offset the Cox-2 tendency to clot blood. Wouldn't you know it? Daily aspirin doses cause exactly the kind of stomach upset the Cox-2 inhibitors were formulated to prevent in the first place!

That's not, however, the last word on the dangers of these inhibitors. According to the June 2001 issue of the prominent medical journal *Lancet,* they may also trigger kidney failure in some cases. Kidney failure and ulcers are also well-known and sometimes lethal side effects of the most commonly taken arthritis drugs, NSAIDs (nonsteroidal anti-inflammatory drugs), such as aspirin and ibuprofen, known more commonly by brand names like Advil and Motrin. Dr. Garret A. FitzGerald of the University of Pennsylvania School of Medicine and his research team published a study in the *New England Journal of Medicine* (Dec. 20, 2001) reporting that taking ibuprofen at about the same time as taking aspirin may cancel out aspirin's blood-thinning effects. This is bad news for heart and stroke patients.

To further complicate matters, the FDA detials in a recent issue of the *Archives of Internal Medicine* five cases of aseptic (nonbacterial) meningitis that are believed to be associated with the use of Vioxx. The victims, ranging in age from 16 to 67, all developed sysmptoms within as little as 12 days after starting the drug—and all ended up hospitalized with this life-threatening disease. And a recent Associated Press story reported that at least six other cases of meningitis have been linked to Celebrex.

Remicade and Embrel, two other name-brand medicines used for a number of rheumatic conditions, are now under scrutiny for devastating side effects as well. An increased risk of tuberculosis in Remicade's case and, according to its own label, an increased risk of multiple sclerosis in Embrel's case are two possible side effects.

Although these numbers are certainly small they point out the very real possibility of severe side effects with certain prescription drugs that are thought to be safe.

The Complementary and Conventional Medicine Partnership

Natural healing, also known as alternative medicine, has been given a new name by the medical world—complementary medicine. Maybe that's because many doctors have finally decided that if you can't beat 'em you may as well join 'em. People everywhere, including doctors themselves, recognize that conventional medicine has its limits, and that the best and most effective healing takes place when individuals participate in their own health care by complementing conventional methods with natural-healing care. In fact, many people begin a natural healing plan as a "complement" to the conventional medicine prescribed by their doctors and then replace it with only natural health care as they reap the benefits and regain their health.

The rewards of adopting a more natural or complimentary approach to treating your arthritis are great. At the top of the list is adding more joy and activity to your life as pain and arthritis flareups are managed more effectively and are better controlled. But the list goes on—by adopting a natural arthritis-management plan, you can at least lessen your dependency on strong pharmaceutical medicines and at the most give them up and live free of their fearsome side effects.

Why a Personalized Plan?
Don't Most Things Work for Everybody?

The one thing that unites arthritis patients and people who suffer from joint conditions is *pain*. Beyond that, people have different pain-tolerance levels, expressions of their disease, and levels of health, responsibility, and lifestyle. This book can provide you with the best ways for managing arthritis and supporting your joints, but it's up to every individual to find out what works best for him or her. And, believe it or not, the path to this discovery can actually be quite enjoyable as you get in touch with your body and learn to control your own health.

See this journey as an opportunity to be adventurous and revitalize the old routine. Try some green tea. Sign up for a yoga class. Go swimming. Meditate every day for at least 10 minutes. Drop dairy products from your diet for a couple of weeks and see if you feel better. Order a tofu dish the next time you do Chinese take-out. Join an arthritis support group to compare notes or start one yourself, even if it's just you and a friend. Make a list of the things you enjoy doing and then do at least one of them every week. Buy yourself some flowers. Attitude is such a big part of controlling this disease that you will be shocked by how empowering some simple changes in your outlook on life can be on your health.

It can be difficult at first to change your lifestyle, find time to exercise, or give up foods you're used to having—but the difficulty and resistance you feel don't last long, especially when the rewards are felt so quickly.

Mind, Body and Spirit—the Components of Your Arthritis-management Plan

Your personal arthritis-management plan should be as individual as you are. However, it should include the following basic components:

Using your mind

Maintain a positive outlook and cultivate your mind's ability to reduce stress and heal. Manage your pain through the power of your mind, by using methods like visualization and meditation.

Helping your body

Follow a healthy, arthritis-busting diet and an effective exercise program, along with bodywork techniques that promote relaxation and healing.

Fulfilling your spirit

Do the things you enjoy, be with the people you love, and participate in activities that inspire you. Remember attitude can make the difference between a pain-filled day or a pain-free one.

Don't Wait Until Tomorrow—Start Right Now

Here are two simple exercises to get you started and inspired. They provide a good introduction for learning how effective your mind can be when it comes to reducing tension in your body. They work so quickly and effectively for some individuals that they are sometimes referred to as the parlor tricks of pain management. Give them a try. You might be surprised by how well they work for you.

Using Your Mind to Relax Your Body

Since the early 1970s, when biofeedback caught the public's interest, the connection linking mind, body, and health has been thoroughly researched and substantiated. For years, positive thinking, meditation, visualization, and other mind/body techniques have helped to quicken the path of healing for those suffering from everything from cancer to burns. These same techniques can be used to improve the lives of those suffering from arthritis as well, particularly in terms of stress reduction, pain management, and the prevention of flareups.

One of the first steps in reducing stress is learning to relax. One method, known as progressive relaxation, teaches you to become aware of the tension in your body and then how to let it go in order to relax.

Try this simple exercise for stress reduction. Sit or lie down in a comfortable position. Begin to concentrate on your toes—not on any of your problems of the day or on your pain. Tell yourself that your toes are relaxed. Believe that your toes are relaxed. You might want to imagine a relaxing warmth spreading over your toes. Once you have felt the tension leave your toes, concentrate on your feet. Work up the body from there, to the ankles, calves, thighs, and so on, relaxing your body as you go. Do not move too quickly and do not move on to the next part of your body until the one you have been concentrating on is fully relaxed.

This exercise may sound almost too simple to be effective, but it works wonders for many people. You will get better at it with practice—so if it doesn't work right away, give it some time. Once you have mastered it, you will discover that you not only feel more relaxed but also can better cope with the situations that arise in your daily life.

Varieties of this technique, utilizing creative visualization, have successfully been used by arthritis sufferers to reduce pain. For example, people with Reynaud's syndrome, a condition that causes decreased blood flow to the fingers (or other extremities) and skin color to change when one is exposed to cold, have been able to successfully raise the temperature in their hands by concentrating and visualizing that they are holding something warm or that their hands are immersed in warm water.

Perhaps your arthritic pain is causing your knee to feel as if a hammer is pounding on it. To try the creative-visualization technique out on your own, try visualizing that hammer is hitting your knee. Once you have that image firmly imbedded in your mind, visualize the hammer slowing down. It is now hitting your knee less frequently, and eventually it stops completely. For some people, this type of visualization exercise can lessen and even eliminate the pain. Again, remember that these techniques may take some practice to master.

Another helpful pain-control technique, one that most moms will recognize, is deep breathing. When you become excited or agitated, your breathing often becomes tight and shallow.

Controlled deep breathing can help you relax. Close your eyes and visualize being in a beautiful place or doing something you enjoy. Slowly inhale through your nose until you cannot take in any more air. Hold your breath briefly. Then exhale slowly through your mouth. Repeat this three more times. Then breathe normally. This simple exercise can help relieve the tension in your body, a common trigger for pain.

Now that you're more relaxed, read on to learn how changing your diet can affect your arthritis symptoms.

• CHAPTER 3 •

Eating for Joint Support and Pain Management

"Let food be your medicine." A wise man, centuries ago, spoke that memorable phrase. References to this ancient concept can be found in the Old Testament as well. It's an idea that has stood the test of time. Unfortunately, as society progressed, we turned away from the natural healing practiced by our ancestors and turned to synthetic medications, thinking they were much better.

But now modern science is proving that this ancient concept is much wiser than we had ever thought possible. Foods, legendary for their healing properties, are once again being used, researched, extracted, combined, and promoted as a means for helping people retain or restore their health. Indeed, more than ever, it would be the wise person who lets food be his or her medicine. And this is especially true for those struggling with the pain of arthritis.

Our joints, our bones, and our muscles cry out in pain when denied the nutrition in fresh, wholesome foods that they need to maintain, heal, and revive. It's little wonder that unwholesome eating habits, often compounded by food sensitivities and an unhealthy weight, can wreak havoc on the bodies of those suffering with arthritis.

The good news is that many arthritis patients experience near miraculous pain reduction, renewed mobility, and increased vitality when they follow a diet void of processed foods and rich in natural ones.

The Diet That Promotes Disease

It's not unusual to find that those afflicted with arthritis consume too many foods made from refined flour, too many sweets, and too many saturated animal fats and hydrogenated oils. For the most part, when analyzed, the typical arthritis patient's diet (and the typical American diet for that matter) is overwhelmed with refined carbohydrates and lacking in fiber, vitamins, and minerals. The damage to the joints due to this pattern of eating does not appear overnight but surfaces after many years.

Cartilage was previously thought to be fairly inert matter, but it's anything but. It repairs, heals, and renews itself. A proper diet and proper nutrition can support that process. If you are afflicted with arthritis, the damage that poor eating habits may have contributed to it can be reduced if you eliminate or severely restrict your intake of refined carbohydrates and other health-robbing processed foods.

Obesity and Arthritis

If you ask any rheumatologist, or any health-care practitioner for that matter, he'll agree that one thing that most of his patients don't understand is this: After the age of 20, you must cut back a little on calories (i.e., the amount of food you eat) for every decade you live. Our metabolism naturally slows down as time goes on, and only by eating less and eating healthy (along with engaging in moderate exercise) can we stave off the extra weight and degenerative health conditions that so often come with the years.

Medical doctors have been aware of the connection between obesity and an increased incidence of osteoarthritis for some time. For a long time, however, they could not say for sure if obesity caused arthritis. The extra weight on the joints, it was clear, aggravated the condition. For this reason alone, patients were (and are) encouraged to lose it.

Some researchers now believe that obesity may, indeed, cause arthritis. Scientists at Boston University followed 1,420 participants in the Framingham (Massachusetts) Heart Study over 30 years. They found that people who were overweight when the study began were more likely to develop osteoarthritis than individuals of average weight involved in the same study. In fact, the heaviest 20 percent of the women were twice as prone to this condition than the average participant in the overall study. A similar study of more than 5,000 people, as part of the First National Health and Nutrition Examination Survey, drew a similar connection between obesity and arthritis.

David T. Felson, M.D., who worked on both of the research projects, believes that the changes in metabolism due to obesity may influence the onset of osteoarthritis in some people. One of his reasons for this conclusion is the fact that obese people develop arthritis in their fingers and other joints that would not ordinarily be strained by extra weight.

Plain and simple, extra weight on the joints can most likely trigger arthritis and certainly can make the symptoms of it worse. However, if you are overweight and you lose those extra pounds, there's often a significant reduction in pain and flareups, along with increased mobility. Losing weight may be difficult, but the rewards of feeling better are well worth the effort. Losing even a few pounds can put that old spring back into your step.

Getting Started With a Strict, Cleansing Diet

Some alternative physicians will have their patients who wish to alleviate their arthritic condition follow a cleansing diet of only uncooked, fresh foods for two to three weeks. In fact, in severe cases of arthritis, it is not uncommon for an alternative practitioner to recommend that a patient eat such foods for up to eight weeks. Although you can vary a cleansing diet depending on your own particular tastes, the uncooked fresh foods you choose should include a combination of the following:

- fruits
- vegetables
- nuts
- seeds
- spring or filtered water

If you choose to try a fresh-food cleansing diet, experts recommend that you also abstain from coffee, black tea, alcohol, nicotine, and sweets during the diet as well. The elimination of these items may help to remove toxins, reduce synovial effusions, and eliminate the fluid in the soft connective tissue of the joints. This diet can also strengthen the normal functioning of the body tissues and increase the body's potassium reserve. Eventually, the "rest" this diet gives your body can allow your nervous system and endocrine glands to recover.

Many experts believe that the typical rheumatic patient's blood flows sluggishly because of the clotting of the red cells that stems from low body energy. A raw-food diet can often increase overall energy which may help combat this condition.

After the two- to three-week period, whole grains, vegetable broth, and potatoes boiled in their skins (preferably red potatoes, because they contain less gluten) can be added back into your diet. If, with these foods, you continue to see improvement in your condition and experience no negative reactions (such as an increase in pain or swelling), you may add cooked vegetables, whole-grain breads, and small quantities of unsalted butter. Once these foods have been reintroduced into your diet without your experiencing any problems, you may then add mild white cheese, cottage cheese, and yogurt.

Cleansing diets have been used safely for hundreds of years to restore health. Countless numbers of people have had positive results using them. Adopting one might just be the ticket to living a pain-free life. A big bonus of the cleansing diet is that it can also reveal hidden food sensitivities you may not have been aware you had.

Hidden Food Sensitivities

As unbelievable as it may sound, a great deal of your arthritis pain could be a direct result of what you eat. The chances are very high that several of the foods you eat on a daily basis are *trigger foods* that cause subtle—but serious—immunological reactions in your bloodstream.

Hours or even days after you eat those trigger foods, you may experience fatigue, headaches, digestive problems, insomnia, skin breakouts, and **joint pain**, but you may never connect those symptoms to the foods that cause them. This is a phenomenon known as hidden food sensitivity—and it affects a large number of people who suffer from arthritis.

When you have a sensitivity to certain foods, your body is unable to thoroughly digest the food and process the nutrients it contains. As a result, incompletely digested food particles pass through the digestive-tract walls and into your bloodstream. They are eventually deposited in tissue, where your white blood cells can mistake them for foreign bodies.

> **T I P**
>
> By keeping a chart for several weeks of what you eat and when you experience pain, headaches, or fatigue, you may be able to uncover if you have any hidden food sensitivities.

Your immune system then mounts an attack against these *invaders*, just as it would against a virus, bacteria, or even a cancer cell. Your system is flooded with histamines, prostaglandin, and other immune chemicals. These chemicals can be extremely irritating to your tissues, causing pain and inflammation. This natural body-defense system is also the reason a bout of flu or a case of extreme food poisoning, such as salmonella, can leave you terribly stiff and sore. If this condition is left untreated, permanent damage to the joint tissue can occur.

From Rapid Aging to Rejuvenation: A Success Story.

Linda faced her 50th birthday, only a few months away, with overwhelming sadness. In the previous five years, she felt as though she had aged 20 years or more. A former athlete, she was tired all the time, carried an extra 20 pounds she couldn't seem to lose, and instead of greeting the day with her former zeal woke up wracked with pain after a poor night's sleep. She got out of bed limping and figured she had full-blown arthritis that would only get worse. Her bad digestion sent her to a gastroenterologist, who added acid blockers to her daily regimen of over-the-counter painkillers.

Through a friend's encouragement, Linda summoned her determination and went on a strict personalized cleansing and elimination diet. For one month, she gave up dairy products, wheat, sugar, fruit (because of its sugar content), and red meat, eating mostly vegetables, some whole grains, and fish. She substituted green tea for black tea and coffee, drank more water, and added a tablespoon of flaxseed oil to her diet. After a month, she added fruit back into her diet, along with a few fermented dairy products, namely yogurt and kefir.

Immediately, the extra pounds began to drop off and her energy increased. She felt well enough to join a spa and begin exercising. Furthermore, to her great joy, her digestion improved so much that she was able to cut back and eventually give up medication, knowing it would stay that way as long as she followed her healthy diet. Best of all was the seemingly miraculous elimination of pain. For Linda—for now and maybe forever—arthritis is not a part of her life. In her own words, "I didn't realize as I got older how allergic I had become to so many foods. I didn't realize the toll they were taking on my health. Without these foods, I feel better and younger now than I have in a decade. I was very sick, but now I feel as if I have my life back."

Digestive Enzymes—the Missing Link

Boosting digestive enzymes through a natural, whole food diet reduces and reverses food sensitivity in the following way: These enzymes decrease the number of undigested and partially digested food particles entering the bloodstream. This, in turn, prevents the immune reactions that lead to digestive and joint discomfort.

To increase your intake of enzymes naturally, try to have raw foods make up 20 percent to 25 percent of your diet. You may not think of items like cereal, crackers, bread, and milk as "cooked" foods, but all of these are processed at temperatures that can destroy the enzyme content. Obviously, all canned fruits and vegetables have been heat-processed; even frozen vegetables, however, are unlikely to contain large quantities of natural enzymes. Although freezing does not destroy enzymes, most frozen vegetables are blanched in boiling water before freezing.

Raw, unprocessed foods like fresh fruits and vegetables, uncooked grains, and raw nuts and seeds contain active enzymes. Naturally fermented foods like sauerkraut, yogurt, kefir, miso, tempeh, and tamari sauce are also rich in enzymes. Consuming sprouted grains and seeds will increase both the enzymes' activity and the nutritional value of these foods.

A Permanent, Health-promoting Diet

Several months on this diet, in the great majority of cases, reduces arthritic pain and the disease's other often-crippling symptoms. It also supports joints in their effort to reduce inflammation and repair themselves. For long-lasting freedom from arthritis, though, you should continue to avoid processed foods and keep your diet rich in fresh, natural foods; raw fruits; vegetables; and nuts. In fact, these foods should compose roughly one-half of your total intake of food. The other half should be made up of whole grains, cooked vegetables, lightly cooked potatoes, and dairy products.

Red meat should be eaten only on rare occasions. Instead, substitute poultry or fish. The essential fatty acids of fish, in fact, are extremely valuable to the body's joints and to your overall good health.

Before we discuss further the types of foods and nutrients that can help to strengthen and support your body, you should be aware that there are a few common foods—namely nightshades, meat, tobacco, and carbonated sodas—that may be negatively affecting your joint health.

Shedding Some Light on Nightshades

For years, eliminating a group of commonly eaten vegetables called nightshades was gospel in the natural treatment of arthritis. Nightshade vegetables include potatoes, tomatoes, eggplant, peppers, and tobacco (chewed or smoked). Arthritis patients are often encouraged to eliminate them from their diet, because they contain substances that can block enzymes in one's muscles from properly metabolizing waste materials.

It is true that for the vast majority of people eating nightshades poses no problems, which is why eliminating them is not as universally promoted as it once was. But for those that may have a sensitivity *and* suffer from arthritis, stopping the consumption of nightshades **can** greatly reduce flareups.

According to Dr. Norman F. Childers, who documented the connection between these foods and arthritis, the problem is one of toxicity—a type of slow poisoning. These foods release toxins that initiate the stimulation of solanine, a crystalline alkaloid that festers in the joints and muscles. With time Dr. Childers says, this substance lowers the body's resistance and prompts the onset of arthritis. Even though only about 5 percent to 10 percent of the general population has an actual sensitivity to nightshades, Dr. Childers' research indicates that more than 70 percent of arthritis sufferers found relief when abstaining from these foods: That's certainly a compelling reason to try eliminating them from your diet to see if your symptoms improve.

Experts suggest eliminating all nightshades from your diet and keeping a record of your arthritis pain for at least three weeks and up to four months. If you find that your symptoms are reduced or disappear during that time, you probably do have a *sensitivity* and should permanently eliminate nightshades from your diet.

A NIGHTSHADE ELIMINATION SUCCESS STORY

One person helped through the elimination of the nightshade family was a gentleman who had been bothered for 20 years with arthritis. As he eliminated potatoes, tomatoes, eggplant, and peppers from his diet and stopped smoking, the painful daily realities of the disease disappeared. The man explains:"For a time, I could not believe what was happening to me. It simply couldn't be that easy. But, in just three months, the pain and restricted movement from 20 years of arthritis were gone! And it happened *without a single aspirin.*"

More About Tobacco

The toxic effects of tobacco do not stop with your lungs and heart. Tobacco appears to trigger the development of arthritis. The *Annals of Rheumatic Diseases* reported in 2001 on a study that compared over 200 rheumatoid-arthritis patients to a control group of people without the disease. Results showed that there were significantly more smokers among the rheumatoid-arthritis sufferers and that most of them had no family history of the disease. The results caused researchers to speculate that tobacco can play a role in the development, or aggravation, of arthritis in some people.

Arthritis and Meat Consumption

Current research is showing that there might be a connection between eating large amounts of meat and experiencing symptoms of arthritis. In fact, it turns out many arthritis sufferers are *also* big meat eaters. By contrast, a lower incidence of arthritis is found in vegetarians. Although a definite connection has not been confirmed between meat eating and arthritis, as is the case with nightshades, researchers strongly suspect it exists. Many people report that a reduction or even an elimination of their symptoms occurs when they reduce the amount of meat in their diets.

The possibility of a meat and arthritis connection has been explored by scientists for more than 11 years now. The prestigious medical journal *Lancet* reported in 1991 on a study in Norway that involved 27 rheumatoid-arthritis patients. These patients were put on a strict whole-food vegetarian diet for a year. Instead of showing an expected progression in their disease, the outcome showed a significant decline in tender and swollen joints, less pain and morning stiffness, increased strength, and overall improvement.

These findings were backed up by another study, reported upon in the *British Journal of Nutrition*, which followed the diets of 44 rheumatoid-arthritis patients for over a year. The conclusion? Those patients on a vegetarian diet had fewer symptoms and flare-ups than those who ate meat and other animal products.

A coincidence? Hardly. Red meat contains between 20 and 50 times more phosphorus than calcium. Phosphorus stimulates the parathyroid glands, responsible for the mobilization of calcium that forms the bones. Leeched from bones, where it belongs, this calcium is then available to be deposited around the joints, leading to arthritic conditions and pain. This is why substituting tofu, legumes, nuts, fish, and poultry for red meat is a step in the right direction for arthritis patients. Your heart will thank you for it, too.

A second possible source of excess phosphorus is carbonated soft drinks. Eating less meat and ending your consumption of carbonated soft drinks while adding calcium and magnesium supplements to your daily routine can make a significant difference in your arthritis symptoms.

Most physicians recommend between 800 and 1,000 mg of calcium and 400 and 800 mg of magnesium daily. It is extremely important to take these two minerals together, as they are bound together in the body. There are tablets available that contain both of these essential minerals in the proper combinations. They can be found at your local health-food store, grocery store, or pharmacy.

> ### T I P
>
> When you eliminate foods from your diet for health reasons, be patient about results. Sometimes it can take three to four months to notice a real improvement. But time passes quickly whether we take charge of our health or not, and a period of several months, once behind us, is not such a big deal after all, especially if the payoff is feeling great!

Healing, Regenerative Oils

A friend of mine was riding down the highway when he noticed smoke pouring out of his car engine. After he had his car towed and checked out, the mechanic told him what was wrong. "All the oil leaked out," the technician said, "and your engine blew. It's ruined. You might as well buy a new car."

An engine—any type of engine—cannot run without the proper oil. It needs lubrication to keep all the gears and other complex parts running smoothly and efficiently. The human body is very similar to an engine in this respect. While the body does not literally blow up, as a car may, it does, indeed, manifest the damage through one or more degenerative diseases (such as heart disease and arthritis). Unlike the case with a car, however, we cannot run out and buy a new body once the damage has occurred.

What Kind of Oil?

When we say the human body needs more oil, we do not mean that people should indiscriminately consume all types of oils and fats. Only certain kinds are required and are beneficial. In fact, consuming the wrong kinds of oils and fats, such as saturated and hydrogenated oils, can be detrimental to your health. The right oils, used sparingly, provide your body with nutrients and essential fatty acids required for good health.

Essential Fatty Acids (EFAs)

The essential fatty acids found in unrefined, cold-pressed vegetable oils are important for promoting overall good health as well as for combatting or preventing arthritis. Both linoleic (omega-6) and linolenic (omega-3) fatty acids are vital to life. They also contribute to the prevention of a build-up of plaque in the arteries.

Fatty acids serve to transport oxygen throughout the body. Every cell requires oxygen. Each organ of the body needs it to function properly. When the membranes surrounding and protecting the cells have this oxygen, harmful bacteria cannot enter.

Essential fatty acids also control chromosomes during cell division and are necessary to the formation of new cell membranes once the cell has divided. Because we know that cancer cells are abnormal cells that grow and perpetuate themselves by division, it is easy to understand why essential fatty acids may be extremely important not only as a preventive measure but also as a form of treatment. (For more information on this topic, see *How to Fight*

Cancer & Win, by William L. Fischer, Agora Health Books, Baltimore, MD.)

Deficiencies May Be Widespread

Many health authorities are only now beginning to realize that deficiencies of essential fatty acids may be more common than previously thought. Research demonstrates that the tissues and blood levels of those suffering from degenerative diseases, such as

---

IS YOUR BODY DRYING OUT?

Dry skin and other areas of dryness on your body may be signals of a lack of proper dietary oils in your diet. While this doesn't mean you have arthritis, these symptoms *may* mean that the drying-out process, which can often precede the development of arthritis, may already be taking place in your body. In fact, these signals may precede the onset of an arthritic condition by five to 10 years.

- dry, cracking, or inflamed joints
- stiffness upon rising in the morning
- numbing or tingling sensations in the extremities
- cold or clammy hands and legs
- dry skin on different parts of the body
- dandruff
- brittle or splitting fingernails
- etch markings on the teeth
- dry, scaly ears and absence of earwax
- encrustation in the corners of the eyes
- premature graying of the hair
- the development of wrinkles
- the development of varicose veins
- bleeding gums
- loss of color or change in complexion

---

arthritis, lack essential fatty acids. When the diet is lacking in these all-important substances, serious health problems develop. Many "diseases of civilization," such as cancer, heart disease, and arthritis, are fostered by an excessive intake of saturated fats and chemically altered fats. These are void of any essential fatty acids.

Saturated fat, hydrogenated oils, and partially hydrogenated oils may have started with the full complement of fatty acids necessary for good health, but the processing system used to prepare them for consumption destroyed any nutritional value they had. Furthermore, essential fatty acids are fragile substances and are easily destroyed in the heating process used to create many of our common vegetable oils.

Flaxseed (Linseed) Oil

One of the best oils is unrefined, cold-pressed flaxseed (also known as linseed) oil. It contains high levels of linoleic **and** linolenic acids, valuable substances in the formation of prostaglandin.

Perhaps that is an unfamiliar term to you, but prostaglandins control many processes related to our metabolism. They are continuously produced by many cells and released into the bloodstream to do their work. They affect the cardiovascular system and are present in the lungs, kidneys, pancreas, prostate gland, and brain.

There are more than a dozen important prostaglandins, and all are them are formed from essential fatty acids. If your system is not getting these fatty acids, it cannot produce the prostaglandin it needs for healthy metabolic functioning.

So what does this have to do with your arthritis? A lot! Many experts now see arthritis as a metabolic condition, a dysfunction of the body's metabolism. Arthritis is a drying up and eventually a damaging of the body's joints. Most experts agree, also, that the breakdown process begins with the cartilage of the joints.

With the proper oil, according to many research reports, the cartilage can be lubricated via the nearby joint cavity. The oils, in this manner, are filtered into the cartilage and provide it with extra elasticity, which keeps it from wearing out.

Flaxseed Oil as a Therapeutic Agent

In its unrefined form, flaxseed oil contains both linoleic and linolenic (better known as omega-6 and omega-3) fatty acids. In fact, of all vegetable oils, flaxseed's percentage of these essential fatty acids is the highest at 72 percent. See page 53 to compare the percentages of these essential substances in other oils.

> LOW-FAT, NOT ZERO-FAT DIET
>
> Even if you are on a strict, low-fat diet, be sure you have at least 1 teaspoon daily of oil rich in essential fatty acids. It can make all the difference in your overall health and well-being.

If you decide to add flaxseed oil to your diet because of its many health benefits, start with a tablespoon a day at most. Many people find that this is all they need to make a difference. Be careful to use only *unrefined and cold-pressed* flaxseed oil, and keep it refrigerated. This method of processing ensures that the essential fatty acids and other nutrients won't be destroyed, as happens when oils are heated to extreme temperatures. In particular, you should *never* cook with flaxseed oil but instead add it cold out of the refrigerator. If the label on the flaxseed oil you buy does not say that the oil is unrefined and cold-pressed, don't buy it. Flaxseed oil, bottled or in capsules, may be found in your local health-food stores in the refrigerated cases. Be sure to check the expiration date before purchasing.

Many people are puzzled about just how they should add flaxseed oil to their daily routine. Following are some simple suggestions for adding a spoonful of flaxseed oil to your diet:

- mix it with cottage cheese and some chopped green onions or salsa
- mix with cottage cheese, berries, and almonds
- add it to vegetables
- blend it into juices
- mix it with lemon juice and use it as a salad dressing
- take it in capsules

Although flaxseed oil provides both omega-6 and omega-3 essential fatty acids, other oils rich in linoleic (omega-6) acid are the safflower, canola, sunflower, corn oil, and, to a lesser extent, olive varieties. The formation of prostaglandin requires both omega-6 and omega-3 fatty acids. Since most vegetable oils other than flaxseed are rich solely in omega-6, you can supply your body with needed omega-3 by eating cold-water ocean fish, an excellent source of omega-3 essential fatty acids (See page 55.)

Following are the essential-fatty-acid values of some of the more popular polyunsaturated oils: Check the chart on the next page to see how your favorite type of oil compares with the others.

Cod-liver Oil

Long a folk remedy for a variety of ailments, cod-liver oil is another oil that can benefit the arthritis sufferer.

For several years now, scientists at Cardiff University in Wales have been researching the effects of cod-liver oil on joints and cartilage. Previously, they found that the omega-3 fatty acids in cod-liver oil could actually "switch off" or reverse the action of the enzymes that degrade collagen and break down cartilage. Current research suggests that taking cod-liver oil may prevent the development or progression of arthritis as well as relieve its symptoms.

Cod-liver oil may also be particularly effective for the arthritis sufferer because of its high vitamin D content, which is necessary to stimulate calcium absorption. It should be used carefully, however, as an excess of vitamin D, although a rare occurrence, can be toxic to the body.

Experts say that, for maximum effect, you should take a little cod-liver oil mixed with orange juice three to four hours after your

---

Unrefined, cold-pressed flaxseed oil is being used therapeutically by many European physicians and alternative medicine practitioners who are treating the following conditions:

Conditions	Benefits
arthritis	promotes healing
age-related complaints	improves many common deficiencies
arteriosclerosis	reduces cholesterol and triglyceride levels
cancer	helps to fortify the immune system
eczema	aids all skin disorders
bronchial spasms	reduces the severity of the spasms
swollen prostate gland	reduces swelling
intestinal complaints	regulates activity
stomach ulcers	normalizes gastric juices
immune deficiencies	boost's the body's immune system

evening meal. Fresh-squeezed orange juice is best, as it does not contain the preservatives, additives, and unnatural sugars of many commercial brands.

Squeeze half an orange and strain the pulp. Place 2 ounces in a glass along with 1 tablespoon of cod-liver oil. Stir well for 30 to 45 seconds. You will notice the formation of tiny bubbles. Drink immediately.

You can drink this mixture either three to four hours after your evening meal or in the morning. If you choose to drink the mixture in the morning, you only need to wait 1 1/2 to two hours before eating—the stomach empties more quickly in the morning.

	Linoleic acid (omega-6)	Linolenic acid (omega-3)
flaxseed	14%	58%
safflower	75%	—
sunflower	65%	—
corn	59%	—
canola	24%	10%
olive	8%	1%

If you wish, you may also take the oil with milk. This may be an excellent choice for those who experience arthritic-related deformities in their joints. According to some specialists, such deformities indicate an allergy to citric acid or fruit sugar.

After several months of supplementing your diet with cod-liver oil, you may find that the "drying-up" process that has been occurring throughout your body is reversing itself. Many users notice an improvement in dry skin or scalp. When this occurs, you may *gradually* reduce the amount of cod-liver oil you take. See "Is

Your Body Drying Out?" on page 48 for a list of the symptoms of the "drying-out" process.

Eventually, you may only need to take the oil every other day. Let your body be your guide. When you see improvements, try the every-other-day dosage for about three months. Then, if you continue to feel good you may reduce the frequency to every other week—which will then be your permanent maintenance dosage.

Those who have diabetes, high blood pressure, related heart disease, or gallbladder problems should take the cod-liver oil and orange-juice blend only every other day or even twice a week, because their bodies cannot assimilate oils as efficiently or as quickly. Those with diabetes, of course, must also be careful about the amount of orange juice they drink, due to its high sugar content. If you have any of these conditions, talk to your doctor before adding cod-liver oil to your diet.

If, in addition to having arthritis, you also have an ulcer, dermatitis, eczema, psoriasis, or any other skin disorder, you may not want to use orange juice. These ailments may indicate an allergy to citric acid, fruit sugar, or both. Instead try mixing your cod-liver oil with milk.

If you use the cod-liver-oil and orange-juice mixture and experience any sort of discomfort, discontinue use. You can instead try taking the oil with milk or alone in capsules.

Cold-water Ocean Fish

Have you ever driven through a coastal town and seen a sign or bumper sticker that read "Eat Fish, Live Longer"? That popular bumper sticker speaks the truth. Fish contains an abundance of omega-3 essential fatty acids, and among them is eicosapentaenoic acid (EPA). EPA, according to a fast-growing mountain of research, is critical in alleviating the symptoms of arthritis and those of numerous other health conditions.

EPA is used by the body to manufacture prostaglandin, the substance that helps to reduce inflammation. Cold-water ocean fish are an excellent source of EPA and should be included as a frequent part of your permanent diet.

COLD-WATER OCEAN FISH:
anchovies
cod
flounder
halibut
herring
orange roughy
salmon
sardines
sea bass
tuna

If you don't eat red meat, poultry, or dairy products, you still might consider eating some salmon. If the bears of Alaska can eat 24 whole salmon a day, you can probably eat a few ounces once or twice a week. Although fresh food is always best, if you don't like the taste of fish, or simply prefer the convenience, you may opt instead to take advantage of the omega-3 capsules now available. Even conventional doctors are recommending these supplements to some of their heart patients, because they appear to help fight off a variety of cardiac related problems. (See William L. Fisher's *How to Fight Heart Disease & Win*, Agora Health Books, for more information on this subject.)

Enzyme-rich Fruits and Vegetables Fight Arthritis

To fight arthritis and restore good health, your diet should consist mainly of nutritious fruits and vegetables. Consider the fact that animals, which later turn up on your dinner table as steaks, pork chops, or roasts, get their cell-building power from vegetables, grains, and other plants. When you eat meat for protein, as most people do, it is almost like you are getting a second hand source for cell-building. Balance your diet by eating plenty of raw, fresh fruits and vegetables.

Most ailments, including arthritis, respond to the curative powers found naturally in fresh fruits and vegetables. Vegetables give us vitamins, salts, trace elements, chlorophyll, and yeast without fouling our bodies with wastes and toxins.

Fresh fruits and vegetables are excellent sources of fiber. The walls of the cells of vegetables are actually made of fiber, which is indispensable to the human digestive system. Fiber works in the intestines like a cleaning machine, sweeping their walls. Vegetables are among the champions of fiber. If you were able to check the nutritional balance of food on a scale by putting meat, sugar, salt, fats, and white flour on one side and fresh fruits, raw vegetables, honey, and whole grains on the other, the scale would lean heavily toward the second group. The first group is full of wastes and toxins and poor in vitamins, enzymes, trace elements, mineral salts, chlorophyll, and fiber—all the healing riches you receive when you choose foods from the second group.

To protect the body's organs from excessive fatigue, aging, and illness, it is wise to choose raw vegetables as often as possible. Cooking vegetables inevitably causes them to lose some of their nutrients. Eat intelligently and choose your foods carefully. Buy only the freshest vegetables and fruits. Never soak your vegetables in water, a common mistake, which causes them to lose many of their beneficial minerals. Instead opt for washing them just before eating.

Some of the fruits and vegetables that are especially effective in helping arthritis patients regain health are lemons, raspberries, grapes, currants, apples, pears, tomatoes, leeks, green beans, onions, carrots, and celery. Many folk remedies recommend eating onions and grapes; they are believed to inhibit the production of uric acid, which can lead to gout.

Eat Your Carrots

Herbalists suggest that people suffering from arthritis should have an abundance of carrots in their diet—in any form: raw, grated, or juiced. Although researchers have not yet uncovered an exact reason why, this vegetable has been shown to diminish the pain of both osteoarthritis and rheumatoid arthritis as well as that of gout in some cases.

One of the theories behind the apparent pain-relieving properties of carrots revolves around the wealth of vitamins they contain. They are, of course, already well known for their high vitamin-A content; there are, however, a number of other beneficial nutrients in carrots as well, including the B-complex vitamins and vitamins C, D, and E. Vitamin C is essential for the proper development of connective tissue, which is vital to healthy joints.

It is best to eat carrots raw or drink raw carrot juice, because, as is always the case with vegetables, cooking them destroys much of the vitamin content. If you find that you can't munch on whole, raw carrots because they are too difficult to bite—grate them. But don't grate them in advance and store them. The vegetable loses much of its nutrients by sitting. In whatever form you choose to eat your carrots, you should make sure they are as fresh as possible.

Some experts believe the specific nutrients in carrots stimulate the endocrine glands and protect the nervous system. These same nutrients will also help to provide your body with energy. And if you feel more energetic, you will be more likely to engage in some type of physical activity, which is, of course, a great therapy for those suffering with arthritis.

Juicing

A popular and healthy method of consuming fruits and vegetables these days is drinking juices made from fresh produce and prepared in a home blender or juicer. Fruits and vegetables should always be at room temperature before being made into juice drinks. Drinking fresh homemade juices is a delicious way of providing your body with many of the nutrients essential to beating arthritis.

Although fresh, whole fruits and vegetables contain valuable fiber, nothing beats freshly squeezed fruit and vegetable juices for a concentrated dose of activated enzymes. Consider getting a juicer and adding one or two glasses a day of fresh juice to your diet. Go wild with your vegetable juices, blending health-boosting cocktails that include some of these nutritious arthritis-busting vegetables:

| celery | parsley | spinach | carrots |
| beets | tomatoes | onions | |

The Internet, any good bookstore, or a library can provide you with scores of delicious juice recipes, or you can invent your own!

Preparing Fresh Vegetables

When preparing raw, fresh vegetables, which are extremely important in the first several weeks of your new diet, you should follow these four basic rules:

1. Vegetables should be eaten as fresh as possible. It is best to use organic vegetables whenever you can. Additionally, they should be prepared just before

eating—not only to avoid wilting and loss of fluids but also to retain as high a vitamin content as possible. Do not shred or chop vegetables until you are ready to eat them. They lose their nutrients when they sit in the open air.

2. High quality is essential. Leafy and root vegetables should be young and tender, with little bruising. The higher the quality of the vegetables and fruits, the better the vitamin content. This, of course, translates into a better diet and more health benefits for you.

3. Clean your vegetables thoroughly to remove any possible contaminates.

4. Choose well-balanced combinations. Each meal of raw vegetables should, if at all possible, consist of one red vegetable, one yellow one, and one green one. A therapeutic diet, such as this one, should also include plenty of green, leafy vegetables.

Arthritis Vanishes – A Case Study

An 8-year-old boy who suffered from severe rheumatoid arthritis was put on a vegetable-and-fruit-heavy therapeutic diet similar to the one I have outlined here and is now living symptom-free. "His arthritis had spread to every joint of his body before I had him placed on the therapeutic diet," his mother explained. "Billy was in the hospital almost four months out of every year."

Billy's mom continued, describing the side effects that her son experienced from his various medications. "He developed stomach ulcers, internal bleeding, and allergies."

But when he began eating differently, his symptoms not only

eased but eventually disappeared. "He has thrived," reports his mom. "There are no more ulcers, no more allergies, and, best of all, no more visible arthritis. He is now able to gain weight for the first time since he was 5 years old. His weight never was more than 30 pounds. He now weighs 54 pounds."

"The change in Billy was so remarkable that his teachers did not recognize him when he returned to school from summer vacation. And, best of all, he no longer takes any medication at all."

Success stories like Billy's are not uncommon for those who are able to commit to a therapeutic diet like this one. Although everyone cannot expect the same dramatic effects that Billy experienced, most people's overall health and well-being will be improved. Healthy eating sets up a good foundation for overall good health.

Chili Peppers

"That'll clear your sinuses!" Whenever you hear that expression, chances are somebody is talking about chili peppers. Folklore claims that a drop or two of hot-pepper extract can help everything from colds to conjunctivitis, in addition to having the ability to kill off intestinal parasites. Chili peppers have traditionally been used to treat arthritis and with a reportedly high success rate. Science has finally revealed the reason why chili peppers work so well.

Researchers have now found the neurological mechanism by which capsaicin suppresses pain. The active ingredient in chili peppers, and in cayenne, is *capsaicin*, which stimulates and then desensitizes the "warmth detectors" in the hypothalamus gland. This substance induces a reduction in the nerve cells of a neurotransmitter called Substance P, which relays pain sensations to the central nervous system. In effect, capsaicin short-circuits the perception of pain.

Chili-pepper extract is being tested as an analgesic (pain-killer). A single injection of capsaicin has been shown to ease certain kinds of chronic pain for weeks, according to research conducted by Thomas Burks, Ph.D, chairman of the pharmacology department of the University of Arizona Health Services Center in Tucson. Dr. Burks is optimistic that capsaicin will eventually be used as the basis of a drug to alleviate the pain of arthritis naturally.

But you don't need to wait until capsaicin is available in an injectable form to benefit from its pain-relieving effects. Capsaic in capsules and even ointments is widely available in health food stores. Merely rubbing an ointment of capsaicin on the skin has been shown to numb pain. Many chili-pepper enthusiasts also swear by the peppers' ability to fight pain and increase your pain threshold when eaten.

If you want to benefit from the natural medicinal qualities of chili peppers but are not normally a hot-food fan, try following these tips:

1. Eat a little bit of hot food at a time. Just about everyone can build a tolerance for hot, spicy food. You might even learn to love it. Just start out slowly!

2. Start with mild chili peppers and slowly build up to hotter ones.

3. Quench the burning sensation with cool yogurt or cottage cheese. Native Americans always traditionally eat something cold with chili peppers to ease their fiery bite. And anyone who enjoys those hot dishes from India knows that they are often served with a cooling yogurt sauce.

Experts suggest that those suffering from arthritis take two capsaicin capsules three times daily with a glass of milk or apple juice. At the onset of this therapy, you may notice a slight increase in your pain; this, however, will soon diminish. It is important that you take these capsules on a regular basis to build up a certain level of capsaicin in your system and to enjoy the lasting benefits.

It's also important to note that chili peppers appear to have the ability to lower blood-sugar levels. While this is good news for diabetics (some health-care professionals suggest three capsules of capsaicin daily for diabetics), it is distinctly bad news for those who suffer from low blood sugar or hypoglycemia. Hypoglycemics are counseled to stay away from any foods or supplements with capsaicin without consulting with their doctors first.

Green Tea – Enjoy a Cup or More Every Day

Taking a tea break with a delicious cup of green tea not only is relaxing and enjoyable but also offers a big bonus for your health. Green tea's antioxidant properties that help fight cancer and heart disease have received significant notice in the press. Much lesser known is its anti-inflammatory properties that are so valuable to arthritis patients.

According to a 2001 issue of the *Journal of Nutrition*, green tea contains gallic acid, which is the basis for its anti-inflammatory and thus soothing effect. A study by the National Academy of Sciences found that green tea reduces arthritic inflammation in laboratory animals by up to 50 percent.

It used to be that one could find green tea only in Asian restaurants, but today the tea is readily available in grocery stores and health-food stores everywhere. Although the caffeine level of green tea is lower than that of black tea, you can buy a decaffeinated version if you prefer—as well as a variety of fruit-flavored and spice-flavored blends.

Take a tea break at least once a day. Sip leisurely and take advantage of your green-tea break to slow down and take a few deep breaths. As you will find out in Chapter 5 and Chapter 6, relaxation is an integral part of your overall plan for beating arthritis.

Feeling Better – What a Concept!

As you progress in your new whole-food eating plan, you will find yourself encouraged by the almost immediate improvement in your health. As the days progress, your diet and food choices will increase and you will become more in tune with your body and how it reacts to the foods you put into it. You might be surprised by the enthusiasm you start to feel for this new healthy lifestyle. The time will probably come when you won't be able to imagine living without your new eating plan and the accompanying spring that it puts back into your step.

• C H A P T E R   4 •

Natural Relief With Nutritional Supplements and Herbs

It wasn't too long ago that healing with vitamins and herbs was considered useless by mainstream medicine. My, how times have changed! Today, many doctors and other health-care practitioners recommend both vitamins and herbs to their patients for arthritis and a wide variety of other ailments. This chapter takes a look at the most prominent supplements and herbs used to alleviate the symptoms of arthritis, as well as some of the traditional herbal treatments that have stood the test of time.

Vitamins and Nutritional Supplements

Healthful eating plus a good multivitamin with minerals (taken daily) will go a long way in fighting off the aches and pains of arthritis. Along with a healthy diet and a good multivitamin, there are a number of supplements and herbs you might want to consider as part of your regular arthritis-busting routine. Keep in mind that nothing works for everyone. Still, with some patience, you might find one or more nutritional supplements that work perfectly for you.

Vitamin E

Doctors used to be baffled by the ability of vitamin E to relieve the pain of arthritis, but they now recognize that it may have a lot to do with vitamin E's antioxidant properties. Antioxidants "scavenge" and help the body eliminate free radicals. Free radicals are dangerous to our health. These sickness-causing molecules attack healthy tissue. Vitamin E prevents this from happening and in doing so helps to prevent the degeneration of tissue caused by arthritis, as well as relieve inflammation.

Vitamin D

Vitamin D, the "sunshine" vitamin for strong bones, plays a role in preventing the progression of arthritis. In one study, scientists at the Boston University Medical Center studied the development of osteoarthritis in the knees of 556 people over a two-year period. Lower levels of vitamin D were consistently found in those patients who suffered the greatest progression of arthritis, and those with above-average levels of vitamin D were shown to be least likely to develop arthitits in the knee. Researchers concluded that vitamin D probably slows down the progression of osteoarthritis.

Low blood levels of vitamin D and a low intake of it have been linked with osteoarthritis. Low levels of this vitamin can also result in bone weakness, leading to fractures and in turn raising one's risk of developing osteoarthritis. However, getting a sufficient amount of vitamin D can reduce cartilage damage in people with osteoarthritis and may decrease the severity of rheumatoid arthritis.

A protective daily dosage of 400 IU is recommended by most experts. Do not, however, exceed 1,000 IU daily, because vitamin D can build up in the liver and become toxic if taken in excess. Mineral oil, alcohol, and some anticonvulsant therapies can interfere with the amount of vitamin D you are getting.

Vitamin C

Good old vitamin C seems to be good for just about everything. Well, arthritis is no exception. This nutrient is essential in the maintenance of the strength and proper functioning of the body's tissues. Vitamin C helps to build and repair collagen, the main building block of cartilage.

One doctor who uses vitamin C treatments for his arthritis patients explains as follows: "We take arthritics that are practically crippled and give them their health back. Even the worst cases are rehabilitated in six months."

He prescribes 10,000 mg of oral vitamin C daily, having his patients build to this amount slowly. At first, they take one 500-mg tablet with each meal and before going to bed. They stay on this dosage for several days. The doctor then gradually increases the amount taken until his patients are taking five tablets (2,500 mg) four times daily. The physician also noted that as large as these doses are, very little of it is unneeded and gets dumped unused into the urine.

One study that confirms this need for vitamin C for arthritis sufferers shows that those afflicted with this disease appear to be deficient in or have low levels of vitamin C. If you take more vitamin C than your body needs for normal functioning, the excess is eliminated through the urine. This dumping will not occur, though, until the tissues throughout the body are saturated with the nutrient. A healthy person's tissues may reach this saturation point with as little as 200 mg per day. In some people, though, especially arthritics, this point may not be reached until 15,000 mg have been taken.

It should be noted that large amounts of aspirin tend to use up vitamin C more rapidly. Aspirin usage may have contributed to the findings by two researchers in Ireland who confirmed that vitamin-C deficiencies are not uncommon in arthritis patients. Scientists at Trinity College in Dublin, Ireland, demonstrated that those with rheumatoid arthritis sometimes require larger amounts of vitamin C in their diets than do healthy folks. They measured vitamin C levels in a group of healthy people and a group with rheumatoid arthritis. Of those in the arthritis group, a full 85 percent had levels that were well below normal. In fact, the level of vitamin C level was so low in these people that they qualified for a diagnosis of subclinical scurvy!

> ### TIP
>
> Talk to your doctor or other health-care practitioner. Keeping him or her informed of your progress and any nutritional supplements you may plan to take is very important, so that prescription and over-the-counter medication can be appropriately adjusted or reduced as symptoms change. Don't expect your doctor to ask about your use of complementary medicine (few do) but tell him or her about it anyway.

If you find it difficult to obtain enough vitamin-C through your diet, you may want to consider taking a supplement. There are several excellent brands currently on the market. We advise you to consider taking one that also contains *bioflavonoids.* The bioflavonoids heighten the powers of the vitamin.

Vitamin P, or Bioflavonoids

In 1753, Scottish naval surgeon James Lind proved that scurvy, at the time the leading cause of death of seamen on long voyages, could be prevented by providing fresh fruit to the sailors. However, the reason *why* this worked was still a mystery—as vitamin C was still an unknown and unnamed substance. In fact, it wasn't until the late 1920s that Dr. Albert Szent-Gyorgyi, a Hungarian physician and scientist, succeeded in isolating vitamin C from oranges.

Most authorities were satisfied that vitamin C was the active element in citrus fruits. Dr. Szent-Gyorgyi continued his laboratory work and, in 1936, won the Nobel Prize when he discovered a group of additional elements in fresh lemons and green peppers. When these newly isolated elements were given to patients, long *with* the vitamin C they were taking, the patients responded more favorably than when given vitamin C alone.

These elements, eventually named flavone glycosides, or bioflavonoids, together were named Vitamin P. The P refers to the strengthening effect these elements have on the permeability of the capillaries, the tiniest blood vessels. So far, researchers have identified rutin, hesperidin, and citrin as bioflavonoids, but there may be more.

Although many fresh fruits and vegetables are good sources of bioflavonoids, they are largely destroyed by cooking. It is in the white pulpy part of raw vegetables and the thin skin separating the sections in citrus fruits that you find bioflavonoids. In nature, vitamin C and vitamin P are found together and work synergistically in the body. Each activates the other, and together they are more powerful than either one alone.

Bioflavonoids increase the strength of the capillaries. Like vitamin C, they are water-soluble and readily absorbed from the gastrointestinal tract into the bloodstream. They exhibit no toxicity, and any excess is excreted through urination and perspiration. Results of clinical tests on the preventive and therapeutic uses of bioflavonoids have been published in respected medical journals worldwide. Because many infections and certain degenerative conditions, such as arthritis, are associated with weakened capillaries, the effects of bioflavonoids are especially important.

Rose hips are an extremely rich source of bioflavonoids and contain 30 times more vitamin C than oranges. Many experts recommend a rose-hip supplement for increasing both your vitamin C and your bioflavonoid intake. Rose hips may be purchased powdered or in tablet form at most health-food stores.

The results of a randomized, controlled trial on the use of rose hips as a therapy for arthritis sufferers was published in the June 2001 issue of *Gesundheitswesen*, a German medical journal. Researchers found that there was a significant decline in pain for those on the rose-hip therapy, as well as a measurable improvement in the flexibility of the affected joint. They concluded that rose hips do indeed have anti-inflammatory properties and that although more research is needed to identify exactly what elements in rose hips are responsible for the positive results, they should be considered a useful treatment for arthritis.

Citrus fruits, grapes, plums, currants, apricots, cherries,

BIOFLAVONOID THERAPY, A CASE STUDY

Dr. James R. West of the Morrell Memorial Hospital in Lakeland, Florida, used bioflavonoids to treat a woman in her middle 50s who was suffering from rheumatoid arthritis. The woman was afflicted with arthritic pain in her hands, wrists, elbows, knees, ankles, and right shoulder. After two weeks of the bioflavonoid therapy, the pain had all but been eliminated and her blood pressure dropped to a healthy 136. After five weeks, her joints were moving more freely and she had a great deal more stamina. The story of Dr. West's patient is only one of many success stories.

blackberries, green peppers, and both black and green tea are all excellent sources of bioflavonoids. Keep in mind that there is 10 times the concentration of bioflavonoids in the edible part of a fruit than there is in only its juice.

Vitamin B₅ — Pantothenic Acid

Pantothenic acid, also known as vitamin B₅, may help to reduce the pain and stiffness of arthritis.

Studies confirm that pantothenic-acid levels are lower in those suffering from arthritis than in healthy individuals. One study demonstrated that arthritis sufferers found relief from their painful symptoms when given injections of 50 mg of calcium pantothenate daily (which is 500 percent of the established U.S. recommended daily allowance).

Another study, performed with oral supplements of the nutrient, produced equally impressive results. Researchers found that that oral calcium pantothenate could significantly reduce the duration of morning stiffness, the severity of pain, and, perhaps most significantly, the degree of disability an arthritis patient experienced. Doses administered in this study began at levels of 500 mg daily and were gradually increased to 2,000 mg.

The current U.S. recommended daily allowance for pantothenic acid is 10 mg. Dr. Roger Williams, who is credited with discovering this nutrient, considers this number to be far too low. Despite this, experts estimate that most Americans receive only one-half to one-third of the current *minimum* guidelines.

Calcium

Calcium's role in building and protecting bones and cartilage is well documented. Its role in preventing broken bones and thus heading off osteoporosis and osteoarthritis is clear as well.

Most people, especially women, in the United States do not get enough calcium in their diets. To further complicate matters, steroids, which are commonly prescribed to control the inflammation associated with arthritis, prevent the body from properly absorbing calcium. This situation can sometimes lead to severe calcium deficiencies, bone loss, and osteoporosis. However, researchers at UT Southwestern Medical Center in Dallas have recently determined that taking calcium and vitamin D *together* aids in the absorption of the calcium and in some cases can halt and even reverse the bone loss.

Other substances, such as salt, phosphorus (found in some soft drinks), sugar, saturated fat, caffeine, and aluminum-containing antacids, can cause you to lose calcium. It is wise to limit the amounts of these items in your diet.

Calcium is available in a variety of forms. High lead content has been found in some types however, so you should be cautious when choosing a calcium supplement. Choose a name brand you recognize. The two most popular and widely available types are calcium carbonate and calcium citrate. Calcium citrate is most easily used by the body and easy to digest. Calcium carbonate is also safe and is often a little less expensive than the citrate form. Experts say that adults 19 to 50 need about 1000 mg of calcium per day. After age 50, that should be increased to 1,200 mg each day. Never exceed 5,000 mg of calcium in a day and do not go above 2,000 mg for a significant period of time. Large doses of calcium can lead to kidney stones or other serious health problems.

Calcium can be obtained through a number of foods including cheese, almonds, bok choy, Brazil nuts, broccoli, cabbage, greens, sardines, yogurt, caviar, dried figs, and oysters. It can also be found in a number of herbs and spices, including basil, cinnamon, dill weed, fennel, ginseng, kelp, oregano, poppy seeds, and sage.

The Calcium/Magnesium Connection

Magnesium is critical to the proper absorption and utilization of calcium. This mineral is a part of what makes up your teeth and bones. Although magnesium is plentiful in nuts, seeds, unrefined whole grains, legumes, and vegetables, the typical American diet is sorely lacking in these foods. Large amounts of sugar and alcohol, also typical in the American diet, can cause magnesium to be dumped in the urine. And poor soil quality means that the magnesium that was once available in our foods has been diminished.

If you decide to supplement your diet with magnesium, look for a supplement that is marked "soluble" on the label; that means that it will be easier for your body to absorb. There are a number of acceptable types of magnesium supplements, including magnesium citrate, magnesium gluconate, and magnesium lactate. A typical recommended dosage for adult men is 400 mg to 420 mg per day. Experts usually recommend that adult women supplement with 310 mg to 320 mg per day. There are a number of supplements on the market that combine your daily calcium and magnesium requirements into one pill.

Zinc

The essential trace mineral zinc is one most people associate with reducing cold and flu symptoms, but studies show it might also help with your swollen joints. One such study demonstrated that zinc could be valuable in treating the joint pain, swelling, and stiffness of rheumatoid arthritis. The study divided a group of arthritis sufferers into two smaller groups. The first group was given zinc supplements, while the other received a placebo. During the 12-week period of the study, those receiving the zinc supplement began to feel better. Their swelling diminished, they walked faster, and their morning stiffness lessened more quickly than before.

Another study, conducted in Denmark, demonstrated that a zinc supplement allowed arthritis patients to reduce the amount of painkilling medication they needed. In addition, their joints were less swollen and were more flexible after supplementation with zinc.

We absorb about 20 percent to 40 percent of the zinc that is in the food we eat. The zinc found in red meat, fish, and poultry is generally better absorbed than the type found in vegetables, dairy products, and eggs. The best sources for the more usable form of zinc are oysters, shrimp, crab, red meat, and other shellfish.

There are several different kinds of zinc supplements available. The most common type is zinc sulfate. It is less expensive than other forms but is not easily absorbed and can cause stomach upset. Other forms of zinc are zinc picolinate, zinc citrate, zinc acetate, zinc glycerate, and zinc monomethionine. Too much zinc can be toxic, so don't ever exceed 50 mg a day. Many multivitamin or multimineral preparations contain a reasonable amount of this mineral.

Boron

If you take a multivitamin or multimineral preparation, be sure it includes at least 3 milligrams of boron. A major study compiling demographic data showed a clear connection could be drawn between countries that had low amounts of boron in the soil and higher incidences of arthritis. According to Dr. Rex E. Newnham, there has been a sharp rise in the average number of people with muscolo-skeletal disease in countries with boron-deficient soil. He points to Jamaica and Mauritius as examples of countries with low levels of boron in the food supply and higher than average incidences of arthritis.

The work of the U.S. Department of Agriculture confirmed the importance of boron to good bone health when it demonstrated that within only eight days of supplementation with a daily 3-mg dose of boron (a dose considered acceptable by most experts) a test group of postmenopausal women lost 40 percent less calcium, one-third less magnesium, and slightly less phosphorus through their urine. These three minerals are essential to building bone and maintaining bone health.

Boron can be obtained naturally in a number of foods. Check the chart below to see which foods have the highest levels of it. (These numbers are averages, since boron content can increase or decrease depending on the levels available in the soil in which

FOODS WITH THE HIGHEST LEVELS OF BORON

(in ug (micrograms*) / g (grams) fresh weight)

soy meal	28 ug
prunes	27 ug
almonds	23 ug
rosehips	19 ug
peanuts	18 ug
hazel nuts	16 ug
dates	9.2 ug
honey	7.2 ug
wines	8.5 ug
raisins	2.5 ug

*1000 micrograms = 1 milligram

foods are grown.)

Royal Jelly

Royal jelly has been called "nature's richest health food," and it has been reported to help ease the pain and discomfort of arthritis in some people.

You may not be familiar with royal jelly. It literally is the food of honeybees, and scientists believe that it is what allows a queen bee to be created in a hive. Bees—all of them—feed on royal jelly, a type of liquid similar to milk, for the first four days after they are hatched. After four days, however, the supply is cut off to all but the queen bee. Researchers now have determined that it is the royal jelly diet that gives the queen bee her distinct size and superiority over the worker bees.

Royal jelly is jam-packed with nutrition. It contains all of the amino acids essential for human health plus 10 additional vitamins and six minerals.

There is a good deal of anecdotal evidence (see Janet M's story) for royal jelly's ability to relieve arthritic pain. Some researchers feel it may be the high pantothenic-acid content that gives it its pain-relieving properties. The pantothenic acid may be acting as an anti-inflammatory agent to reduce pain and stiffness in the joints.

If you would like to give royal jelly a try, check with your local health-food store. Carefully read the label of the brand you select to make sure it has not been heated, since heating destroys some of the nutritional content. Any quality brand will clearly state on the label how the supplement was processed.

Warning: If you suffer from a bee allergy, you should avoid royal jelly and other bee products. If you develop

---

ROYAL JELLY—WINNING THEM OVER ONE SUCCESS STORY AT A TIME

Janet M., 57, had been an arthritis sufferer for several years. In that time, her condition had gotten steadily worse. Some days were better than others, of course, but there were some days when it felt as if every bone in her entire body hurt.

One day, Janet went into a local health-food store to buy some vitamins. She casually mentioned her arthritis to the clerk. "Oh yes, I used to be bothered something terrible with joint pain," the clerk commented, "but not anymore." "Since I've been taking royal jelly, I hardly ever complain of arthritis aches and pains," she told Janet.

Curious, Janet bought a bottle of royal jelly capsules. She took them faithfully for several days. In that time, she noticed a slight improvement. It encouraged her to continue. Her husband scoffed at her, but Janet soon became convinced of royal jelly's effectiveness. She found it easier to get out of bed in the morning. Her joints hurt less, and she accomplished more during her day. Within several weeks, even her husband admitted there was a difference in her personality. She was more cheerful and more optimistic about life. "I never would have thought that something that came from a beehive could be so beneficial to people," Janet said.

---

hives, an itchy throat, headache, wheezing, or skin flushing while taking a bee product, you may have an allergy and should discontinue your use of that product immediately.

Propolis

Another treatment many arthritis sufferers report success with comes straight out of the beehive as well. *Propolis* is the resinous substance gathered by the bees from leaf buds and tree bark and used to construct and repair their hives. Propolis is rich in amino acids, as well as the trace elements iron, copper, manganese, and zinc. It contains a wide variety of vitamins including pantothenic acid, which, as I have already mentioned, can act as an anti-inflammatory agent.

The medicinal properties of propolis have been recognized and used for centuries, especially in the treatment of wounds and inflammations of any kind. In fact, in Russia during World War II, it was successfully used to treat battle wounds. It has been used to treat a variety of other conditions as well, including inflammations of the throat and mouth, tonsillitis, and ear infections.

Propolis appears to have anti-inflammatory properties, which would account for its success in treating the symptoms of all types of arthritis and rheumatism. It is often recommended by alternative practitioners for any condition involving harmful bacteria, germs, viruses, or inflammation.

If you want to try supplementing your diet with propolis, you might want to try your local health-food stores as well as online Interent sources. Again, do not use propolis if you have any type of bee allergy, and if you feel any allergic symptoms while taking propolis, you should stop using it immediately.

Apple-cider Vinegar and Honey – A Popular Folk Remedy

In the New England states, it is said that the use of apple-cider vinegar and honey as a treatment to help relieve the painful symptoms of arthritis is as old as—if not older than—the United States itself. The use of both vinegar and honey in medicine has its roots even further back.

Vinegar is a natural germ killer and has been used for centuries in this capacity. It has been said that as far back as 400 B.C. Hippocrates was using vinegar preparations to treat his patients.

Ancient Assyrian medical texts refer to vinegar as a recommended treatment for ear pain. And during the U.S. Civil War, nurses and doctors turned to it as a reliable disinfectant for wounds.

Vinegar is nutritionally dense, with at least a dozen minerals, over half a dozen vitamins, a number of essential acids, and several enzymes. Phosphorous and calcium, two important bone-building elements, as well as potassium and iron, can be found in vinegar.

Like vinegar, honey has been used to disinfect wounds and aid in the healing process. It has been credited with having anti-inflammatory properties as well. A quick search of the medical literature makes it clear that honey's reputation has even gone mainstream, with it being used in a variety of clinical settings to treat wounds, promote healing, and soothe inflammation.

A recent review published in the *American Journal of Clinical Dermatology* confirmed honey's potential for healing. Researchers evaluated the vast amount of existing case studies, experiments, and randomized clinical studies supporting honey's effectiveness and concluded that according to the existing biomedical research honey does in fact demonstrate an ability to rapidly clear infection and reduce inflammation.

Why not try adding some apple-cider vinegar or honey to your diet? Both are relatively cheap and simple remedies that may provide you with some relief from your daily aches and pains.

Try some apple-cider vinegar to dress your next salad. You can use the vinegar straight from the bottle or mix it with olive oil and spices of your choice for a different taste and texture.

Honey can be used as a natural sweetener in your tea or mixed into some plain yogurt for a delicious taste treat.

You might also want to give the traditional New England vinegar and honey mixture a try. You can make your own mixes of vinegar and honey (see the box below for the simple recipe) or purchase a premixed brand from your local health-food store, from a food store, or from a reputable website.

NEW ENGLAND APPLE-CIDER VINEGAR AND HONEY MIX

Mix 2 teaspoons of apple-cider vinegar with 2 teaspoons of honey in a glass of water.

* Sip this drink slowly, as if you were drinking hot coffee.

Other Trace Minerals

Ongoing studies have focused on the role of certain trace minerals in preventing arthritis and its symptoms, and, conversely, on how deficiencies may cause an increase in its development or flareups. If you are deficient in one or all of these minerals, researchers theorize that this deficiency could lead to the development of arthritis or an increase in current arthritic symptoms. Supplementing your diet with these minerals, or adding food sources rich in them to your diet, may halt the progression of the disease or ease its symptoms.

Copper – Copper is an essential nutrient that your body needs in relatively small amounts. It is the main element of red blood cells, and it provides energy for the body. It helps to form collagen and is a key component in the makeup of bone and connective tissue. Research has shown that copper may help to relieve symptoms of arthritis. You can add more copper to your diet by increasing the amount of shellfish and nuts you eat.

Folic acid – Folic acid is a water-soluble B vitamin that the cells in your body use literally thousands of times in a day to, among other things, make blood cells, build muscles, and heal wounds. It is an essential nutrient that nine out of 10 adults get too little of. The body is unable to store folic acid for long periods of time, making it necessary to restore it regularly. Folic acid fights heart disease by affecting the body's use and production of damaging homocysteine, may help to ward off certain cancers, fights certain types of birth defects, and is useful in treating arthritic symptoms, in particular gout. The folic acid content is high in green vegetables, beans, whole grains, and orange juice. For those interested in using a folic-acid supplement, most experts recommend 400 to 800 mcg a day.

Manganese – Manganese is a metal found in plant and animal tissue. It is stored in the body in bone and contributes to the formation of more bone, connective tissues, fats, proteins, and blood clotting. It has been shown to have a protective effect for joints during times of inflammation. People suffering from rheumatoid arthritis are often found to have low levels of manganese. Although there is no RDA for manganese, experts agree that 2 mg to 9 mg per day should be sufficient. You can easily obtain this element in foods like pecans, almonds, wheat germ, leafy vegetables, liver, legumes, and dried fruits.

Selenium – Selenium is a trace mineral that the body needs in very small amounts. It can be found in soil and food. It is a strong antioxidant that improves your blood's ability to deliver oxygen, keeps your tissues elastic and firm, and helps keep the retinas in your eyes healthy. The mineral is passed through soil into the foods we eat but has been severely depleted in many parts of the world, including areas in the United States. The current recommended daily allowance for grown men is 70 micrograms. However, expert recommendations may range from 70 to 200 micrograms per day. You can add more selenium to your diet by eating foods typically high in the mineral, such as fish, poultry, meat, whole grains, Brazil nuts, and vegetables.

Additional Nutritional Supplements and Herbs for Natural Relief

While aspirin and ibuprofen are probably the most common over-the-counter pain relievers for arthritis, they are not without their side effects—especially when used in the large quantities some arthritis sufferers need to experience relief. The most common problems encountered by people using these painkillers are stomach irritation and ulcers.

Other prescription pain relievers are often accompanied by a list of their own side effects. Some of these side effects may be relatively minor, such as an upset stomach, but others, although more rare, may be life-threatening. The popular prescription pain-relieving drug Vioxx, for example, was recently linked to several cases of nonbacterial meningitis, which causes an inflammation of the brain and spinal cord. While Vioxx and similar prescription drugs may be effective treatments for your arthritic pain, you owe it to yourself to be informed about the natural treatments that may work just as well for you.

Fortunately, nature has provided us with alternatives that are less harsh and contain few if any side effects. These include herbal teas and supplements derived from nature. Herbalists of generations past valued the medicinal qualities of plants and respected their abilities to bring relief of pain—including the pain of arthritis.

Because each person reacts differently to different remedies, we suggest that you try several different herbs and joint-support supplements to discover the ones that are most effective for you.

Glucosamine and Chondroitin

Certainly the biggest news in fighting arthritis and maintaining healthy joints involves glucosamine/chondroitin supplements.

The positive stories about the combo's ability to reduce joint pain, stop the progression of osteoarthritis, and even build cartilage are piling up, so much so that research to the tune of millions of dollars is being funded by the National Institutes of Health to find out exactly how it works and how well it works. Fortunately, you don't have to wait for the results, because glucosamine and chondroitin, separately or together as a combination supplement, can already be found at your local pharmacy or health-food store.

Both glucosamine and chondroitin sulphate are found naturally in our bodies. Glucosamine is an amino sugar that plays a part in building and repairing torn cartilage. Chondroitin is part of a protein called proteoglycan that helps cartilage maintain its elasticity by drawing vital fluids to the joints. Although glucosamine is also found in a number of foods, the most common source for supplements is seafood (primarily crab and shrimp shells). If you're allergic to shellfish, glucosamine might not be safe for you.

Chondroitin is extracted from the windpipes of cattle. If you choose not to take glucosamine, you can also derive benefits from taking chondroitin alone. The reverse is also true. If you are concerned about taking a bovine-based supplement, you can experience benefits from glucosamine without the chondroitin. (See the sidebar on the next page for information on "mad cow disease"). The fact remains, however, that taking both is still considered most effective for treating arthritis-related conditions, since they support joints in different ways.

Numerous studies done in Europe on hundreds of patients have already shown that a glucosamine and chondroitin combination has an anti-inflammatory effect and that it relieves the pain of osteoarthritis as well, if not better, than daily doses of NSAIDs. Furthermore, it doesn't appear to have any negative side effects. Glucosamine and chondroitin supplements are among the few natural alternative treatments that have jumped the barrier between alternative medicine and mainstream and landed firmly on the mainstream side of the fence. Many doctors have already started recommending the supplements to their patients in hopes that doing so will allow them to reduce their use of strong painkillers.

One recent news report cited a highly respected independent testing group's endorsement of glucosamine/chondroitin as being effective not only in reducing pain but also in rebuilding damaged joints. The report featured one arthritis sufferer who stated that she was in so much pain that she couldn't get out of bed in the morning. After a year on glucosamine/chondroitin supplements, however, she's taking high-impact aerobics. While her results may not be typical, they are certainly dramatic and should call attention

---

MAD COW DISEASE AND CATTLE-DERIVED INGREDIENTS

You no doubt have heard about the fatal brain infection bovine spongiform encephalopathy (BSE), more commonly called mad cow disease. BSE can be passed on to people from infected cows and has been the cause of deaths in several European countries. Understandably, there has been some concern here in the United States regarding supplements and products like chondroitin (extracted from the windpipes of cattle) that are derived from cattle ingredients.

Scientists believe that BSE, which can infect organs and tissues, cannot infect bone or cartilage, since it has no blood supply or nerves that could support the abnormal protein. At this time, the U.S. meat supply is totally free of BSE and there are restrictions on

to the innumerable success stories attributed to this supplement combination.

Research supporting the success behind these supplements continues to pour in. The medical journal *Lancet* reported that glucosamine reduces the pain of osteoarthritis and may possibly indicate a "disease-modifying effect" that points toward a reversal in cartilage loss. In other words, according to this report, glucosamine was found to not only reduce pain, but also, by all indications, rebuild deteriorating cartilage! Even *JAMA*, the *Journal of the American Medical Association*, has jumped on board with its recent favorable review of glucosamine and chondroitin. *JAMA* concluded that glucosamine and chondroitin preparations do demonstrate "moderate to large effects" in combating the pain and joint deterioration associated with arthritis. These are just two examples among scores of studies that are reporting the same positive results.

The combination's benefits, like those of many natural-healing methods, are not instant. Improvement can be seen with consistent and long-term dosage, usually in about 10-12 weeks. Recommended

---

importing any meat or feed from countries that have infected cattle or livestock. In general, the risk of any cartilage products being contaminated with BSE is considered low but does exist.

Experts advise that you never take any supplements made from cow *organs*. If you decide to take supplements containing cow-derived bone or cartilage products, check the label for each to make sure that the ingredients come from U.S. cattle or other countries where no BSE has been found. Since cartilage or bone products *could* possibly be cross-contaminated in the slaughterhouse, the only way to be 100% safe from BSE is to avoid **all** products that are made from animal ingredients.

dosages range anywhere from 800 to 1,200 milligrams each of glucosamine and chondroitin each day. There are a number of supplements on the market that combine glucosamine and chondroitin in one capsule, and they can be found in most drug stores, grocery stores, and health-food stores.

In many countries, glucosamine/chondroitin supplements are available only with a prescription—resulting in strict quality control. In the United States, however, they are readily available without a prescription. As a result, the same quality-control standards do not exist. It's a good idea to get your supplements from a reputable company or chain that prints a toll-free customer-service number on its labels and provides access to a website.

If you are diabetic, it is important to note that some animal studies have shown a possible connection between glucosamine and an increase in insulin resistance. However, these findings have not been replicated in humans and the test subjects in the animal experiments were on continuous high-dosage intravenous glucosamine. If you are diabetic and concerned about how glucosamine may affect your sugar levels, you should monitor your blood levels more closely after starting a glucosamine supplement and stop taking it if your levels increase. You should always, of course, check with your doctor before starting to take any new supplements.

MSM (Methyl Sulfonyl Methane)

Many RA patients swear by the supplement commonly referred to as MSM, saying that it reduces pain and flareups. Although discovered in the early 1980s, methyl sulfonyl methane has only recently had a surge in popularity after arthritis sufferers discovered its apparent ability to ease arthritic symptoms. It has been promoted by actor James Coburn, who has touted this supplement on talk shows as making all the difference in his fight to overcome crippling rheumatoid arthritis.

What is it? MSM is a sulfur molecule found naturally in humans and in many protein foods and vegetables. Sulfur is necessary for maintaining healthy joints, and research shows it may have anti-inflammatory properties. Cooking or processing foods, however, destroys MSM, which is why it's often necessary to take supplements if you want to boost your levels.

In addition to relieving pain and inflammation, MSM is also reported to help stabilize the immune system (which could be helpful for autoimmune disorders like lupus), increase energy, decrease muscle soreness, and reduce allergic reactions. Some users report cosmetic benefits from using MSM, such as an increase in nail toughness and thickening of the hair. Some patients suffering from GERD (a reflux disease) have discovered that taking MSM enables them to reduce their intake of prescription medication.

It is, however, important to note that research on MSM has thus far been limited, with no long-term conclusive studies completed at this time, and its benefits have primarily been reported by word-of-mouth. But that doesn't mean it's not helping the thousands, if not millions, who take it faithfully. It's tasteless, odorless, and considered safe. No toxicity has been reported in connection to MSM. It may, however, have some blood-thinning effects, so be sure to talk to your doctor if you are already taking blood-thinning medication in case your medication needs to be adjusted.

If you're allergic to sulfites, you'll be glad to learn that MSM is not a sulfite but a sulfur compound. Some users may experience a mild upset stomach when using MSM. A typical dosage is 1,000 mg to 3,000 mg daily with meals. Small amounts of MSM are found naturally in green plants, fruits, vegetables, fish, and grains.

SAMe

Like MSM, SAMe (which stands for S-adenosylmethionine) is a naturally occurring substance in the body and has biochemical functions. SAMe supplements are usually made from fermented yeast.

SAMe has primarily built its reputation as a natural antidepressant by raising the brain's levels of dopamine, a substance involved in regulating moods. However, a number of reputable studies dating back to 1987 and a stack of success stories and anecdotal evidence have led to its reputation for reducing osteoarthritic pain and inflammation and improving overall joint function and healing. The consistent use of SAMe has allowed many patients to reduce or replace NSAID painkillers, such as ibuprofen and naproxen. And, unlike such NSAIDs, SAMe does not cause any damage to the digestive tract. It has been available for years in Europe as a prescription medication.

Both folic acid and vitamin B_{12} are necessary to properly absorb SAMe. If, therefore, you decide to try a SAMe supplement, make sure that you have sufficient amounts of them in your diet or daily multivitamin/mineral supplement. Research subjects taking SAMe for osteoarthritis experienced its beneficial effects when using an average of about 1,000 milligrams a day. One study showed a daily dosage of 800 mg per day for six weeks effectively improved symptoms in fibromyalgia patients.

SAMe tends to be somewhat unstable, so be sure to look for packaging that is resistant to air and light—such as enteric coated tablets in foil or blister packs. Do not remove the pills from their packaging until you are ready to take them. A common dosage for osteoarthritis is 600 mg (200 mg taken three times a day) for the first two weeks and then 400 mg for a maintenance dose.

People with Parkinson's disease or those living with bipolar disorder should not take SAMe, because of how its biochemical activity affects the brain. With SAMe, as with all nutritional and herbal supplements, you should talk to your health-care professional before adding it to your diet.

Lyprinol – an Extract From New Zealand Green-lipped Mussels

Medical statistics show that arthritis and rheumatic disorders are almost unknown among the coastal-dwelling Maoris, the native people of New Zealand. Some scientists have theorizing this is true because green-lipped mussels are a major part of their daily diet. According to a centuries-old tradition, the Maoris believe that eating the green-lipped mussel leads to a long and healthy life. Science has now isolated the key ingredient to the health-promoting properties of these mussels—lyprinol.

Lyprinol is a lipid or fat that has been extracted from the New Zealand green-lipped mussel, or Perna canaliculus. Scientists have determined that the anti-arthritic properties attributed to the green-lipped mussel are due to the unique configuration of certain polyunsaturated fatty acids (or PUFAs) called eicosatetraenoic acids (ETAs). Related to the omega-3 fatty acids found in fish and flaxseed oil, ETAs display more intense and targeted anti-inflammatory and antiarthritic activity than any other known PUFA or omega-3 fatty acid.

Research in the 1970s and 1980s confirmed that something in the New Zealand green-lipped mussel had the ability to erase arthritic pain and stiffness. A double-blind placebo-controlled trial conducted in 1980 at the Victoria Hospital in Glasgow, England, tested a powdered mussel supplement on 66 arthritis patients. At the start of the six-month trial, all of the subjects had failed to respond to conventional treatment and were scheduled for surgery to repair badly damaged joints. At the close of the trial, the researchers reported improvements in 68 percent of the rheumatoid-arthritis (RA) patients and in 39 percent of the osteoarthritis (OA) patients. The scientists also noted the low incidence of adverse side effects.

Michael Whitehouse, Ph.D., of the department of medicine at the University of Queensland at Brisbane, Australia, is a recognized authority on drug-action research, with extensive experience with anti-inflammatory drugs and rheumatic diseases. Dr. Whitehouse studied the efficacy of lyprinol by using laboratory animals with adjuvant-induced polyarthritis, which is the closest model for rheumatoid arthritis in humans.

When taken as an oral supplement, lyprinol was able to reduce arthritis-related swelling by a staggering 93 percent to 97 percent. It was also found to be effective when rubbed directly into the affected area. Dr. Whitehouse then compared it to other natural lipids, or fatty acids, known to be helpful in treating arthritis and inflammation. He tested it against flax oil, evening-primrose oil, Norwegian-salmon oil, and MaxEPA (a high-potency fish-oil product). Of these, lyprinol was the most effective in preventing arthritis-related swelling—reducing swelling by 79 percent. MaxEPA was the next best at 50 percent.

However, the real surprise was the dosages used to achieve these results.

In order to achieve a 50 percent effectiveness rate, Dr. Whitehouse used a dosage of 2,000 mg/kg body weight of MaxEPA.

But the effective dosage of lyprinol was only 20 mg/kg—or 1/100 the amount. According to these results, the anti-inflammatory compounds in lyprinol are 200 times more potent than those in MaxEPA (and 350 times more potent than those in evening-primrose oil).

Lyprinol is now being recommended by a growing number of health-care providers to relieve a number of inflammatory conditions, including osteoarthritis, rheumatoid arthritis, and virus-induced arthritis. While lyprinol appears to be a powerful anti-inflammatory and arthritic-pain reliever, it is important to remember that it cannot rebuild or restore previously damaged cartilage.

Lyprinol is available in freeze-dried, ground, or capsule preparations. You should be able to find it at your local health-food store or on the Internet. If your local store does not carry it, they probably can order a supply for you.

For those taking capsules, the most frequent dosage recommendation is 300 mg to 350 mg three times a day. In addition, Dr.Whitehouse's research suggests that rubbing lyprinol into swollen and tender joints can help relieve pain and swelling. To do this, simply open the capsule and squeeze the contents onto the affected area. You should avoid taking lyprinol if you are allergic to seafood or shellfish.

GLA (Gamma-linoleic Acid)

GLA, or Gamma-linoleic acid, is an essential fatty acid found primarily in plants and specifically in black-current oil, evening-primrose oil, and borage oil. Linoleic acid, found in cooking oils and some processed foods, is converted into GLA in the body. Like the health-promoting oils discussed in Chapter 3, GLA can help to relieve pain and inflammation; it may also be specifically effective in relieving symptoms of RA, Reynaud's phenomenon, and Sjogren's syndrome. In fact, human studies show that GLA when taken internally can ease pain and inflammation and has few side effects. Some rheumatoid-arthritis sufferers find that supplementing with GLA allows them to reduce the amount of anti-inflammatory drugs they take.

GLA can be taken in the form of evening-primrose oil, black-currant oil, or borage oil, as well as in capsules. It can also be found added to bottles of cold-pressed flaxseed oil. There is no RDA for GLA. Experts typically recommend 1.4 g per day for arthritis or 1,500 mg to 1,800 mg of oil one to two times a day. Black-currant oil usually contains a higher concentration of GLA then the other oils do.

A number of manufacturing processes can destroy the nutritive value of GLA-containing oils, so be sure to look for a product that is certified as organic by a reputable third party. The brand you choose should be in a light-resistant container, refrigerated, and marked with a freshness date. Check your local health-food or natural-food store; you should find several brands and forms of GLA to choose from.

If you are currently taking any blood thinners, including NSAIDs or herbal supplements, be sure to speak with your doctor before supplementing with GLA, because it may increase their effects.

Shark Cartilage

Shark cartilage, made famous for its anticarcinogenic claims, has reappeared as a healing supplement for osteoarthritis. It is said not only to have an anti-inflammatory effect for many users

---

BEFORE YOU BUY...

A little research can go a long way in making sure you purchase vitamins and supplements from a company that cares about its customers. Toll-free numbers, detailed labeling, expiration dates, company websites, and USP codes are all signs for consumers that the company adheres to quality standards and cares about its reputation. If you have a choice between a recognizable name brand and a brand from a company you don't know, it is probably best to buy from the company that you recognize. That way, you can make sure you're getting your money's worth. Last but not least, take as directed and never exceed recommended dosages.

---

but also, according to some researchers, to be helpful in regenerating cartilage.

Eastern cultures have long touted the health benefits of this substance. In Japan, in fact, shark-fin soup is considered a delicacy and is believed to promote longevity. It was once dismissed by the mainstream as a nonharmful but ineffective folk remedy, but Western science is finally starting to sit up and take notice of the mounting evidence in shark cartilage's favor.

Martin Milner, a naturopathic physician, uses shark cartilage as a natural cancer therapy and has noted its dramatic effect on the arthritis symptoms of his patients. According to Dr. Milner, shark cartilage—in addition to providing chondroitin—offers effective, naturally occurring ingredients not provided by glucosamine or chondroitin supplements alone. These include the following:

- angiogenic-inhibiting proteins, which are substances that prevent additional blood-vessel invasion of the joints in rheumatoid arthritis

- naturally occurring glucosamine and chondroitin for the treatment of osteoarthritis, in forms your body can more easily assimilate

- collagen, which has a body of evidence supporting its efficacy in treating arthritis

- calcium and phosphorus (15% and 7% respectively by weight), both of which are important for maintaining bone health and recommended by the FDA to fight osteoporosis.

All of these substances are vital for cartilage and overall joint health.

Shark cartilage appears to have some significant anti-inflammatory properties. Studies have demonstrated the supplement's ability to reduce pain and inflammation. One recent Canadian study put shark cartilage to the test and found it to be an effective treatment for psoriasis, a condition that can result in extreme inflammation. Experts theorize that it may also be an effective treatment for osteoarthritis, because of its apparent ability to stimulate cartilage to repair itself by delivering cartilage-growth-promoting nutrients to the joints. The substance is also reported to have the beneficial side effect of boosting immunity.

A typical dosage recommendation for the treatment of arthritis is 2,000 mg taken three times a day. Experts suggest taking the supplement on an empty stomach.

Green Tea

Whatever you do, don't wait until your next trip to an Asian restaurant to enjoy a cup of green tea. Start drinking a cup or two at home (and on the job) every day. This beverage, a traditional favorite among the Chinese, has gained quite a reputation for its health-boosting powers. It seems that almost any day of the week there is a headline announcing another study showing green tea's effectiveness in fighting off some illness or disease.

Green tea, which is steamed and dried rather than fermented like black teas, is rich in flavonoids, the pigments in plants that give them their red, blue, and purple colors. Flavonoids are also known for their infection-fighting and antioxidant properties (the ability to scavenge free radicals in the body that cause tissue damage). It's this ability that may make green tea so valuable in fighting arthritis by reducing inflammation and protecting tissue.

In a study by the National Academy of Sciences, green tea added to the diets of laboratory animals with arthritis reduced inflammation by up to 50 percent. Furthermore, signs of immune-system response were markedly lower in the joints of the animals used in the study. Green tea is also cited in numerous studies as helpful for reducing heart disease, cancer, and obesity.

A typical cup of green tea contains about 200 mg to 300 mg of polyphenols (plant-based antioxidants). Experts suggest three to four cups of green tea a day. The tea is now widely available in most grocery stores and can be found in natural-food and health-food stores as well. Green-tea extract is also available, in tablets, capsules, and tinctures.

Do not add any milk-based products to your green-tea, because they can interfere with the action of the polyphenols. If you are sensitive to caffeine, you may want to consider taking a tablet or capsule supplement or trying a decaffeinated brand.

Ginger

Ginger is commonly used in Asian cooking and is also the

primary flavor in the popular soft drink ginger ale. It is thought to be good for just about everything. Considered in Asian medicine to be a *toner*, a substance that promotes overall health and well-being, ginger is also a safe, natural anti-inflammatory and pain reliever.

One targeted study of seven women who were suffering with rheumatoid arthritis found that 5 grams to 50 grams of fresh ginger or capsules containing up to 1 gram of powdered ginger led to less inflammation and joint pain.

You can easily increase the amount of ginger in your diet by trying some Chinese or Indian dishes that feature the hot lemony spice or by drinking natural ginger ales or ginger tea. To relieve the aches and pains associated with arthritis, you can try rubbing ginger oil, available at your local health-food store, directly into the painful joint.

Ginger Tea

Making your own ginger tea is easy. Steep about 2 tablespoons of freshly shredded ginger (available at your local grocery store or Asian food market) in hot water for several minutes. Strain the tea. It is then ready for drinking. Drink two to three cups a day to relieve arthritis pain.

When buying ginger supplements look for ones that contain *pungent compounds* (gingerols and shogaols) to be sure you are getting the most healing benefits. If you are taking any cardiac drugs, anticoagulants, or diabetic drugs, consult with your doctor before increasing your ginger intake.

Club Moss

Club moss is a trailing plant characterized by ramblers that reach out and cling to the ground with small, hairlike roots. These ramblers eventually grow into forked branches.

In addition to helping to fight rheumatism, club moss is said to help relieve the, often excruciating, pain of gout. This natural herbal tea is also reputed to be of benefit to urinary-tract and reproductive organs including the ability to reduce inflammations of the testes.

The tea works so well in relieving painful symptoms for some sufferers that herbalists say one cup a day is all most people need to see a benefit. Club-moss tea is available in most local health-food stores. You should never boil club moss but instead pour hot, never boiling, water over the leaves. Sip a cup of the tea each day, one half-hour before breakfast.

Horsetail

Another tea that many herbalists believe is very effective in treating the symptoms of arthritis is horsetail. A cup daily may eliminate the pain of both rheumatism and osteoarthritis, as well as that of gout. In fact, some herbal specialists believe that this herb is so effective against these conditions that it may actually prevent their development when taken regularly.

Horsetail is rich in silicon, a trace mineral that is thought to be needed in the development and maintance of connective tissues and found in certain bony areas of the body. Horsetail also absorbs calcium, which can then be used by the body to grow bone. The tea is an excellent choice if you suffer from water retention, which can often aggravate swollen and painful joints.

The herb horsetail is also known by various other names, including bottle brush, shave grass, pewterwort, and dutch rushes. This tea is most effective when taken hot. If you like, you may sweeten it with a little honey.

Yarrow

Yarrow, which flourishes in a sunny and warm environment, is a popular European folk medicine. Herbalists often recommend it for inflammation, so it is a natural choice for those suffering from the inflammation and pain of arthritis. Yarrow is a mild diuretic, which may account for some of its abilities to relieve aches and pains.

The plant contains several elements that have been clinically shown to have anti-inflammatory properties. Unlike some of the teas discussed earlier, you may need to drink more than one cup daily to find relief. In fact, you may want to drink three or four cups every day. And to increase the effectiveness of yarrow's natural medicinal powers, try adding a pinch of cayenne pepper to the drink.

Yarrow tea is also effective for easing lower-back pain, bursitis, and just about any menstrual problem. Some herbalists recommend this tea for relief of sinus headaches.

Very large amounts of this plant might interfere with certain blood-thinning or blood-pressure medications. Although it is not likely you would be able to consume the amounts necessary to cause an interaction with any medications you are taking, it is always best to remain cautious and consult with your doctor before adding any supplements to your diet.

Stinging Nettle

Stinging nettle has been used for literally hundreds of years to treat arthritis, rheumatism, and gout. The stinging hairs on the nettle contain irritating chemicals that cause pain when they come into contact with the skin. Stinging nettle in its pure form is known as a counterirritant, meaning that the irritation when directed at a part of the body that is already in pain (such as an arthritic joint) can lessen or dull the original pain. You must be very careful in handling the actual nettle plant and avoid unintended skin contact.

Nettle roots and/or nettle leaves are often used in herbal preparations or teas. Stinging-nettle tea acts as a mild diuretic, helping to relieve pressure on the joints and the pain associated with arthritis. If you are taking drugs for diabetes or low blood sugar, be sure to check with your doctor before trying this tea. The most common dosage recommendation for the tea is to drink about half a cup prior to meals and another half a cup after eating.

Some European herbalists recommend that their patients take stinging-nettle tea with some *Swedish Bitters* (an herbal blend) added. Stinging-nettle tea and Swedish Bitters both can be found in your local health-food store. If your store does not carry them, ask that they order some for you or check the Internet for a reputable mail-order company.

Dandelion

Dandelion, which grows wild in most parts of the world (perhaps even in your own back yard), is rich in vitamins and minerals. The leaves of the dandelion are high in vitamin A and potassium. Dandelion is a mild diuretic which can help to relieve the pressure on swollen or painful joints.

You can make your own dandelion tea of dried or fresh leaves and roots. Simply pour a cup of hot water over 1 to 2 teaspoons of the herb and allow the mixture to sit for about 15 minutes before drinking it. Strain the tea prior to drinking.

Dandelion tea, when taken daily, may act as a detoxifying agent, cleansing the bloodstream of impurities, which according to many physicians may be a contributing cause of arthritis. For best results, drink a cup of this tea a half-hour before breakfast and a half-hour after breakfast daily.

The fresh leaves of the dandelion can also be added to sandwiches or salads or steamed and eaten like spinach. If you choose to pick your own fresh leaves, be sure they come from a protected location that you know has not been exposed to pesticides or other containments.

Feverfew

Feverfew has long been considered a valuable herb by alternative and holistic healers in the treatment of a number ailments, including arthritis. This herb, which bears a flower resembling a daisy, is considered an effective remedy for migraine headaches and perhaps is best known for its ability to relieve this type of pain. But feverfew is also very useful as a natural treatment for arthritic pain. Recent evidence indicates that it may help to prevent the process that leads to inflammation. The active compound in feverfew, a chemical called parthenolide, appears to work by blocking substances in the body that widen and constrict blood vessels and lead to inflammation. The herb also causes the body to slow down the production of the hormonelike prostaglandins that actually cause pain and inflammation.

If you want to try feverfew, be sure that the supplement you choose is made from the herb itself. Also be sure that it contains at least 0.4% of feverfew's active ingredient, parthenolide. A typical dosage is 250 mg of feverfew a day to treat the symptoms of arthritis.

Herbalists caution that feverfew is one of the more powerful natural remedies and, for this reason, should not be used by pregnant women, breast-feeding mothers, babies, or children.

Devil's Claw

With a name like devil's claw you would hardly expect this African herb to be such a blessing to arthritis sufferers. However, countless success stories of those who have given this herb a try attest to its abilities to relieve the pain of arthritis.

Clinical studies have shown that devil's claw is remarkably effective in reducing the pain and swelling of arthritis in rats and increasing the mobility of their joints. According to experts, it is probably effective because of its ability to act as a mild diuretic and a cleanser. Current research indicates that the herb reduces the inflammation by extracting the superfluous fluid from the affected joint areas. This allows the connective tissue to function normally and act as a barrier against toxins. The herb is also reported to be an effective analgesic or pain reliever.

Anecdotal reports and countless succcess stories attest to the pain relief that many have found with devil's claw. One such account is that of a 9-year-old girl, Karen, who was helped by this herb. Karen had a severe case of rheumatoid arthritis, which kept her in constant pain. Her parents had sought all the best doctors and tried everything the medical community had to offer—but she continued to suffer through daily pain. Finally, her parents heard about devil's claw and decided to try it. Within two months, the herb reduced Karen's pain considerably. Today, Karen is able to enjoy life as other children do.

The case of Bertha M., 74, is another devil's claw success story. Bertha suffered from an extreme case of debilitating arthritis, which she developed in her early 40s. For over 30 years, she endured the pain. Her daughter read about devil's-claw bark and decided her mother should give it a try. Bertha, who was in constant pain and desperate for relief, agreed to give the herb a try and embarked on a four-week treatment involving daily supplementation. She later described her improvement as miraculous. "Now my mother is baking cakes and cooking meals and looking after herself once again," her daughter reports.

The devil's claw plant has an extremely long root system. As a native of the Kalahari Desert in Africa, it must survive up to 10 months of drought conditions each year. It is this root that is the valuable portion of the herb.

Some people drink devil's-claw-root tea, but this is a very bitter drink and many cannot tolerate the taste. However, this potent medicinal root is now available in tablet form. There are a number of different brands on the market; some of them, however, are not made from the herb's root, which is the only portion of the plant possessing medicinal qualities. When purchasing this supplement, be sure to choose a brand that is made only from the root.

Devil's claw is considered safe with virtually no side effects. If, however, you have a heart condition or other serious medical condition, check with your doctor before trying devil's claw.

Ayurvedic Herbs From India

Ayurveda is a medical system that has been practiced in India and Nepal for over 4,000 years. The word Ayurveda itself means knowledge *(ayur)* of life *(veda)*. Although Ayurveda has many components, such as diet, exercise, and personal hygiene, herbal medicine is one of its foundations.

Some Ayurvedic herbs may be effective in fighting arthritis with fewer side effects than conventional Western medicines, which is why they are being included with more frequency in herbal formulas for joint support. A number of these herbs, boswellia in particular, have been studied in Europe with positive results and have been used on the Continent for decades.

Boswellia (or Indian Frankincense)

Boswellia is the front-runner for Ayurvedic joint support. It comes from the gummy resin produced by the Boswellia serrata tree. It has been used in Ayurvedic medicine for thousands of years as an anti-inflammatory and to treat osteoarthritis, rheumatoid arthritis, gout, stiffness, and pain.

The acids in the Boswellia plant appear to have anti-inflammatory properties which inhibit the production of hormonelike substances in the body, such as leukotrienes, that cause inflammation. Unlike

---

OTHER AYURVEDIC HERBS USED FOR JOINT SUPPORT:

guggul – acts as an anti-inflammatory

Indian madder – serves as an immune regulator

horseradish tree – acts as a stimulant

gokshura – is a natural steroid that reduces inflammation

musk mallow – supports and helps to maintain healthy joints

guduchi – inhibits bacterial growth and supports the immune system

licorice – stimulates the immune system

---

the case with NSAIDs, use of the Boswellia plant will not lead to stomach irritation or ulceration.

A typical dosage recommendation for treating arthritis symptoms is 150 mg three times a day.

Turmeric

You are probably most familiar with turmeric as a spice found in Indian cooking. It has also been traditionally used to treat a variety of medical conditions, including arthritis.

The active ingredient in this herb, curcumin, has been shown in several studies to lower histamine levels, leading to an overall reduction in inflammation. Other studies have hinted at turmeric's ability to reduce inflammation by stimulating the production of natural cortisone.

Turmeric extracts are available in capsules and tablets, and a typical dosage would be 400 mg to 600 mg three times a day.

Chinese Herbs

Traditional Chinese Medicine (TCM), including herbal formulas and acupuncture (see page 133), has been used effectively for thousands of years. Chinese herbal combinations are often part of the holistic treatment provided by experienced alternative practitioners and acupuncturists. Similar to the theories behind acupuncture, these herbal formulas are primarily directed toward balancing the body's energy and supporting the immune system in order to restore health. Most herbal preparations are created for a specific patient based on the patient's particular imbalances. They can be powerful and healing with few side effects.

TCM is a licensed profession in 27 states, and the National

A WORD ABOUT THUNDER GOD VINE:

Thunder god vine (Tripterygium wilfordii) is a Chinese root used traditionally to treat autoimmune diseases. It is currently being researched as a treatment for RA. At least one study involving RA patients has shown positive results in improving their arthritis. Another study, reported by the Rheumatic Diseases Clinics of North America, said that using the extract allowed 42 out of 100 lupus patients to reduce their daily prescription of prednisone and 12 others to discontinue it. Only an extract from the root of this plant can be used, as the leaves and flowers are toxic and lethal. Thunder god vine may produce a number of varied side effects and should be used with caution and only with the guidance of an experienced health-care practitioner.

Certification Council for Acupuncturists and Oriental Medicine (NCCAOM) administers an annual certification test. An herbalist certified by the NCCAOM will use the title *Diplomate in Chinese Herbal Medicine* (or Dipl. CH NCCAOM) after his or her name. See the resources section for contact information for the NCCAOM and the American Herbalists Guild.

CHAPTER 5

Exercise – Make It Part of Your Life

Pick up almost any book about maintaining good health, retaining mobility and flexibility, reducing chronic pain, managing stress, or increasing longevity, and you'll probably discover that it says the same thing all the others say when it comes to exercise: Do it!

Is it possible to exercise your arthritis away? Well, not quite. But exercise can, in many cases, prevent or delay disability, forestall or prevent surgery, reduce pain, help you to reduce your reliance on prescription medication, and, most importantly, help to fortify your overall health and maintain your mobility and quality of life. If you're thinking, "Well, my arthritis isn't too bad yet, so I can put off exercising," think again. The proper exercise can actually delay the progression of arthritis in a very big way.

Exercise Is the Key to Staying Young

A 60-year-old who exercised regularly all of his or her life can be as fit as or fitter than any younger person who gets little or no exercise at all. Read the stories of those rare individuals who have lived to be 100 years old or more. What is the common thread running through them all? Exercise in some form. It may be that they did physical labor of some type, such as working in the fields, every day of their lives or that they maintained a regular excercise routine.

"But," you say, "I'm already affected by arthritis. I'm not going to live to be 100, and it's probably too late for me to start improving my health." **It is never too late!** You can, indeed, experience the benefits of exercise even if you have a severe case of arthritis. While high-impact sports like jogging and tennis may be beyond you, there are many other kinds of exercise within your reach.

On certain days, when it feels as if every bone in your body is aching, you are probably not very enthusiastic about exercise. If your doctor has ordered rest on those days, rest may indeed be the perfect treatment. But the person suffering from arthritis needs to find a healthy balance between rest and exercise. It is imperative if you have not already developed an exercise program that you do so carefully with the guidance of your health-care practitioner. With arthritis, more than with other health conditions, the right exercise can be good for everything, but the wrong exercise can actually make matters worse by stressing the joints. When designing your exercise program, be sure to keep in mind any other health conditions you may have. If you have a heart condition or athero-sclerosis, you should obviously begin your activities very slowly and increase them gradually.

This chapter reviews several kinds of gentle exercise that are generally recommended for arthritis patients. These include walking, exercising in water, stretching exercises, yoga, Pilates, tai chi, and some deep breathing and relaxation exercises you can enjoy. So take your pick and give those aching joints some support through movement.

Walking

Walking is an excellent exercise. Many experts, in fact, consider it to be the *perfect* exercise, since it is appropriate for almost everyone at any age and at any fitness level. Begin walking for just 10 minutes daily: less if you have difficulties. If you walk outdoors, you have the added bonus of being exposed to sunlight—which stimulates your body's production of vitamin D. This nutrient is essential for proper calcium absorption, an important consideration for arthritis sufferers.

Find a walking buddy to make your daily walks even more enjoyable. Studies show that any exercise program is easier to stick to if you have a workout buddy. You'll be amazed at how quickly your daily walks will add to your sense of well-being. Got a busy day ahead? Park a few blocks away from your destination and enjoy the few minutes it takes to walk there. Walking is a great stress buster, and this gentle form of exercise warms up the muscles

---

WALKING BAREFOOT – A SIMPLE REMEDY

This remedy may seem too simple and too enjoyable to be of much benefit, but many people have found relief with it. Walking barefoot in the early morning grass while it is still wet with dew is one of those delicious pleasures in life we seldom give ourselves permission to do. And, believe it or not, the relief you may be feeling after this activity is not all emotional (though that's an important part of beating any illness, especially those that involve pain like arthritis). Walking barefoot in the wet grass grounds the static electricity in your body and can help to regenerate your energy. After your early morning barefoot stroll, vigorously dry your feet with a rough towel and put on a pair of shoes immediately. If you live in the middle of a city and this remedy is impossible for you to carry out, an energizing alternative it to massage your feet daily with olive oil blended well with 10 drops of pine oil.

---

and can ease the everyday aches and pains of arthritis. If you are feeling sleepy after a big meal, don't lie down on the couch! Get up and walk around the block. In addition to fighting arthritis, it will invigorate you and aid in your digestion.

Aquatic Exercises

Jump in, the water feels wonderful! Exercises performed in water are a great choice for the arthritis sufferer. The water reduces the amount of pressure upon the joints while the exercises are being performed. At the same time, the resistance caused by working against the water helps to build strength. Some YMCAs and local community centers hold water exercise classes specifically designed for those with arthriticlike conditions. Check with your local YMCA or community center to find out if it offers a water-exercise class. It doesn't have to be one designed specifically for

---

A SWIMMINGLY GOOD SUCCESS STORY

George, 56, was suffering terribly from arthritis in his knees. Some days the pain was so crippling that walking just a few feet caused excruciating pain. Outings with his family had become torture, and he often just elected to stay home rather than spoil the fun. One day, his daughter suggested they join the local community pool. She encouraged him by saying that the water would make him feel better. George was doubtful, but he agreed to give it a try. After spending just an hour in the pool, George was a believer! The water relieved the pain of the arthritis in his knees for hours afterward, and he is now going to the pool three to four times a week. "I want to feel exactly how I feel after getting out of the pool **all** the time", George says. His wife reports that sometimes she has to run to keep up with him now and that it has been ages since she replaced the pain relievers in the medicine cabinet.

---

arthritis sufferers; just speak with your instructor before starting the class and explain your special needs. Another good source for information on aquatic classes is your local office of the Arthritis Foundation. The Arthritis Foundation has a water-exercise program called the Arthritis Foundation Aquatics Program (AFAP) that sponsors classes two or three times a week at local pools. The Arthritis Foundation has a local office directory on its website at www.arthritis.org.

While a formal water-exercise class is an excellent and enjoyable option, remember that just about any kind of swimming is beneficial for arthritis patients. If you haven't visited a pool for years, why not go give it a try? Make it a family event and take along the children or grandchildren, or find a swim buddy to share in the fun. You will soon discover the forgotten pleasure of splashing around the pool, and your aching joints will thank you for it. Many arthritis sufferers report hours of relief following a pool visit.

Bathtub Exercises

For those of you who don't feel you are ready for a pool visit, want to add a more gentle form of exercise to your daily routine, or just don't have the time in your schedule for a formal class, there are water exercises that have been designed specifically for those suffering from arthritis that can be performed in the privacy of your home. The exercises I detail here were originally developed by Nancy Kadler, a nationally registered occupational therapist with years of professional experience both in hospitals and in private clinics. These simple exercises, when performed regularly, may help ease the pain of your arthritis and increase your mobility.

Those who are in a severely weakened physical state should limit their initial exercise regimen to only two or three repetitions of the exercises and perform only a small portion of those provided. As you gain strength, you may increase the number of repetitions and add more exercises.

Tips to Get Started

The water temperature of the bathtub or spa should be comfortable enough to allow sore, tight muscles and joints to relax, but not too hot. It is best to start with three repetitions of each activity and slowly increase the number as you begin to feel comfortable. Don't rush your progress. There is nothing to be gained by doing too much too fast. And you may end up causing yourself injury or pain by moving forward too quickly in the hopes of hurrying improvement. Take your time and enjoy the gentle movements and resulting gradual ease of movement.

The following instructions are written with the understanding that you are sitting in your bathtub. If you are using a hot tub instead, you may need to modify the directions slightly. (You also may adapt some of these to use in the pool.)

Foot synchronization: Facing forward, with your legs extended, turn both feet to the right, as far as possible without discomfort. The outside edge of your right foot and the inside edge of your left foot should be resting on or near the bottom of the tub. Now gently rotate both feet in the opposite direction. The outside edge of your left foot and the inside edge of your right foot should end up resting on or near the tub's bottom. Repeat this full rotation once more.

Next, turn both feet inward at the same time so that your big toes touch. Then gently turn them out in the opposite direction, so that your heels are facing each other. Repeat.

Finger swings: Submerge your hands in the tub water, bending your wrists so that the backs of your hands are facing the bottom of the tub. If you cannot bend your wrists this much, bend them as far as you can *comfortably.* Slowly bend your hands upward so that your fingers are pointing toward the ceiling. Do not force your fingers; only bend them as far as is comfortable. Hold this position for a count of three. You should feel some tension through your wrist and forearm. Straighten your hand back out and let your fingers relax. Repeat.

Foot stretches: Sit comfortably in the tub. Bend your knees slightly. Point your toes upward toward the ceiling. Hold for a count of three. You should feel the muscles in your calves tighten. Then, slowly point your toes forward as far as is comfortable. Hold for a count of three.

If you wish, you may also perform a variation of this by pointing the toes of your left foot toward the ceiling and the toes of your right foot straight or away from you at the same time. Hold for a count of three. Reverse the positions of your feet.

You can also try stretching both your hands and feet at the same time for a bit of variety.

Toe holds: Sitting in the tub, bend your knees so that your feet are lying flat on the tub floor. Raise your big toes as high as possible. Your other toes will automatically move. Do not worry about that. Next, curl your big toe and hold it as close to the balls of your feet as possible. Do not lift your feet any higher than absolutely necessary. Again, your other toes will also move.

Thumb cross: Submerge your hands in the water and gently touch your thumbs to your little fingers. Relax your hands. Repeat.

> ### T I P
>
> It's OK if exercise for arthritis patients is a little vigorous or challenging, but it should never be painful. If pain or joint swelling increases during exercise, stop immediately.

Deep-breathing and Relaxation Exercises

Deep-breathing and relaxation exercises are excellent and often underappreciated weapons to add to your arthritis-fighting arsenal. They help to relieve tension, improve circulation, promote the elimination of toxins from the body, and aid in the digestion of food, not to mention their ability to provide your body with increased oxygen, which helps to strengthen and rebuild your health. When you feel relaxed, you are better able to handle life's everyday stressors that contribute to arthritis flareups.

Following are several exercises you can use on a daily basis to help tame the tension. Be sure to find a quiet place without distractions where you can perform these exercises uninterrupted and wear loose and comfortable clothing.

The Breath of Life – Lie flat on your back on a hard surface, preferably the floor. With your mouth closed, slowly inhale deeply through both nostrils. Hold this breath as long as possible. Exhale slowly. Begin with five deep breaths and gradually increase the number you perform until you reach 10. If you cannot perform this five times on your first try, simply do as many as are comfortable and slowly work up to five and beyond. Next, block the left nostril with your finger and perform the same deep-breathing exercise as explained above. Repeat twice. Finally block the right nostril and perform the same deep-breathing exercise as above. Repeat twice.

The Relaxing Release – You may do this exercise sitting in a comfortable chair, lying on the bed, or lying on the floor. Close your eyes, take a deep breath, and hold it. Tighten all the muscles in your body. You should consciously try to think of every single muscle and tighten it as you do. Continue to hold your breath, keeping the muscles tightened for five seconds. After five seconds, let all the air out of your lungs in one quick outward breath and let all your muscles relax completely; allow your body to go limp. Take several deep slow breaths and then repeat the breath-holding and muscle-tensing exercise as described above. Do this complete cycle at least three times.

Progressing with Progressive Relaxation – Sit in a supportive comfortable chair with your back braced against the back of the chair and both feet flat on the floor. You may also lie flat on a firm surface like the floor. Starting with your feet, you are going to alternate between tensing certain muscle groups and relaxing them. Begin by concentrating on your toes. Think about just the muscles in your toes, inhale, and gently tense those muscles. The tension should be firm and deliberate so that you can really feel it, but it should never cause pain or extreme discomfort. If you feel pain or extreme discomfort, stop the exercise immediately. You might notice that it is difficult, at first, to isolate a single muscle group. As you perfect this technique, this process will become easier. Hold the tension on the muscle group for about eight seconds. You may start to feel the muscles shake, which is perfectly normal. After eight seconds, let your breath go and at the same time let all the tension flow out of the muscles to allow them to go completely limp. As the tension flows out of the muscles, imagine any pain flowing out of the muscles with it. Allow yourself to notice the differences between how the tensed muscles feel and how the relaxed ones feel. Relax for about 10 seconds and then repeat the exercise, isolating each set of muscles in your body (calves, thighs, buttocks, stomach, fists, forearms, shoulders, etc.).

You can also try a variation of this progressive-relaxation exercise that involves visualizing a warm, soothing, and relaxing sensation spreading from each muscle group progressively. Just as with the other progressive relaxation exercise I described, you isolate each muscle group, but instead of tensing the muscles, you imagine a soothing warmth entering them, allowing them to relax completely.

Stretching Exercises You Can Do at Home

Following are several simple but effective stretching exercises that are excellent ways to gently warm up and condition your muscles and reduce aches and pains. As with the previous activities, continue with an excercise only as long as it is comfortable. The exercises provided below should not promote pain when performed correctly. If you feel pain as you do any of them, stop. Try the activity again when you feel able, but do not stretch as far. As you become stronger and more flexible, ask your doctor for more exercise suggestions or a referral to a physical therapist, so you can learn more about safely increasing your exercise program.

Be sure that you do all of these exercises slowly. Do not hurry through them and do not try to do them all in your first session in hopes of speeding relief. As always, check with your doctor before starting any kind of exercise program.

The Standing Stretch - Stand with your feet apart. Bend your legs slightly. Clasp your hands behind your back. Very slowly, bend forward from the waist while raising your arms behind your back. Go only as far as is comfortable. When you have stretched as far as your body will allow, hold the position for a count of five. (Do not bounce.) Then slowly reverse the process to return to your original position. Repeat this exercise once.

The Seated Stretch - Sit on the floor with your legs extended straight in front of you. Exhale and then slowly stretch your upper body forward, sliding your hands forward to touch your ankles. Go only as far as is comfortable. If you feel pain, stop. Hold this stretch for a count of five (again, without bouncing). Slowly return to your original position. Perform this stretch three times.

Knee Pulls - Lie on your back with your legs extended straight. Place your hands at your sides. Slowly pull your right leg up toward your chest as far as is comfortable without pain. Grasp the leg with both arms and hold this position for a count of five. Lower your leg to the floor. Repeat the process with your left leg. Repeat this cycle three times.

Next pull both of your legs as close to your chest as possible without pain. Lock your arms around your knees. Hold this position for a count of five. If you can hold it for longer, feel free to do so up to a count of 15. Repeat this once.

Hip Rotators - Lie on your back with your arms at your sides as in the knee pulls. Place your palms down. Pull your knees toward your chest. With your hands on the floor to be used as supports, rotate your hips and legs to the left as far as possible. Your goal is to have your legs touch the floor. You may not be able to achieve this with the first attempt (if ever). Do not become discouraged. It is important that your shoulders and back remain flat against the floor during this stretch to avoid injuring yourself. Reverse your position slowly, bringing your legs toward your chest and then gently placing them back on the floor. Repeat the entire procedure but rotate your hips to the right this time. Perform this exercise two times if possible.

Neck Stretches - Sitting straight, bend your neck to the left as far as you comfortably can. Your goal should be to touch your ear to your shoulder. Don't worry if you are not able to stretch this far (few of us can); only go as far as is as comfortable for you. Bring your head back up to the upright position. Then bend your neck to the right, again going only as far as is comfortable. Repeat this cycle five times.

Next, keeping your head upright, rotate your neck slowly as

far as you comfortably can to one side, back to the center, to the opposite side, and then finally back to the center. Repeat this five times, if possible.

Yoga

People that practice yoga rave about its far-reaching ability to improve their overall health and feelings of well-being from head to toe. And unlike those who favor forms of exercise that may fall to the wayside over the years, yoga fans are often life-long devotees. Most are committed to practicing yoga well into their senior years as a way to retain youth, vigor, and mobility.

The discipline of yoga originated in India, where it has been practiced and perfected for thousands of years. More than simply exercise, yoga is considered to be a holistic health science that promotes the balance of mind and body and the release of one's energy or life force (called *prana*). This balance is achieved primarily by practicing the various yoga postures *(asanas)* and proper yoga breathing methods. The postures themselves, though gentle, provide a complete and satisfying workout, with their emphasis on promoting flexibility, building strength, and encouraging relaxation.

Some people adopt the philosophy and lifestyle of yoga, following its recommendations for eating, selecting clothes, personal hygiene, and spiritual practice. Many simply practice yoga solely as a form of effective exercise.

A decade ago, yoga classes could only be found in big cities; today, however, classes are sprouting up at senior centers, community-recreation centers, and local hospitals. There are various disciplines and styles of yoga, such as hatha yoga, kundalini yoga, and Iyengar yoga. There is even a more rigorous form of yoga called Power Yoga. Some of these yoga classes are taught in a more vigorous manner than others, so it may be best to observe a beginner's class or talk to the insructor before signing up for one. Before you begin the excercises, you should share your concerns or physical limitations with the teacher so he or she can adjust the exercises for you.

There are numerous sources for learning more about yoga, including books, videos, and websites. For beginners, it may be best to take a class so you can get one-on-one help from the teacher and make sure you're assuming the postures correctly. As you begin your yoga class, remember to take it slowly. With consistent practice, you'll progress rapidly and begin to notice the added flexibiity and strength that a regular yoga routine offers.

The Pilates Method

Pilates exercises are also highly recommended for arthritis patients. They are low-impact but vigorous, so they provide a thorough workout without causing further stress to your joints. Each exercise is carefully designed to both stretch and strengthen your body. The Pilates method was created in the 1920s by Joseph Pilates, who used yoga as its foundation. Similar to yoga, the Pilates exercises may help you decrease medication while increasing your flexibility, strength, and sense of balance.

The Pilates exercises have become quite popular, and you can often find a class at your local gym or recreation center. There are also a number of books and videotapes for those who prefer to exercise at home. Be sure to start with a beginner-level program. You can begin the exercises at any age or level of ability and progress from there.

Tai Chi

It seems that every time Western conventional medicine conducts research on the benefits of doing tai chi, this slow and graceful system of exercise, originating from China, scores an A+. Pronounced "tai-chee," this ancient and healing martial art has recently moved into the spotlight as a potential remedy for the pain associated with arthritis. In fact, the Arthritis Foundation, which endorses tai chi for reducing arthritis pain, even used it as the basis for designing one of its most popular exercise programs—which is called range-of-motion (ROM).

Underscoring tai chi's dual role as an effective exercise and therapeutic practice, the National Institutes of Health has credited the practice with the ability to improve balance and reduce the fear of falling in older participants. Many researchers, recognizing the benefits this gentle exercise can offer, have begun to take a serious look at tai chi. At least half a dozen published studies have focused on its role in the treatment of arthritis. One study confirmed marked pain reduction in all 16 arthritis patients who practiced tai chi over a 10-week testing period. Patricia Adler, R.N., who conducted the study, commented that, "Exercises such as tai chi help reduce arthritis pain by increasing circulation and stimulating the repair of damaged joint surfaces. In addition, it stabilizes joint structure by strengthening the soft tissue supporting joints."

Tai chi involves performing a series of slow and controlled body movements while keeping your body upright and straight and controlling your breathing. The exercises may involve stepping, shifting weight, and balancing. It's a low-impact form of exercise that strengthens the body while promoting flexibility, enhancing muscle tone, and improving circulation. In other words, it is perfect for those of us who suffer from arthritis.

As is the case with yoga, the practice of tai chi encourages balancing the body's energy while building flexibility and strength. And even though tai chi is gentle and done slowly, don't underestimate its workout value. Tai chi's fluid movements require concentration and effort. You may even be surprised after your first tai chi session when you find your muscles feel somewhat fatigued; it's similar to the feeling you might get from a more vigorous aerobic workout. There is no age limit for practicing tai chi. In China, in fact, it is not uncommon to see dozens of older folks practicing their tai chi outside in public parks or squares. Once you learn the movements, you can practice them anywhere you go. If you're a beginner, it's best to learn tai chi from a teacher so you can get individualized instruction. There are, of course, videos and books available to help you with the fundamentals if you prefer.

• CHAPTER 6 •

Bodywork and Soothing Topical Remedies

Following a healing diet that includes the appropriate supplements and herbs helps you fight arthritis internally—from the inside out. Exercise, bodywork, and topical remedies are additional ways that you can help yourself naturally—from the outside in.

Following are several external healing methods and topical remedies that can help you feel better by soothing pain away and providing welcome relief and relaxation.

The Healing Qualities of Clay

Clay packs have been used to successfully treat ailments for literally centuries. In fact, clay treatments have been so successful for such a long period of time that it is surprising that relatively few people are aware of their soothing benefits. While current technology has overlooked clay's natural healing properties, this age-old treatment deserves top billing as an effective way to ease arthritis pain.

Holistic and alternative health practitioners report that a

combination of clay and herbs can have lasting positive effects when used to treat arthritis. The clay is mixed into a paste and a hot herbal infusion is added to create what is referred to as a *pack*. This pack is applied directly to the affected part of the body. Clay packs may be applied either hot or cold, depending upon the time of the year and the individual's sensitivities.

You can purchase prepared clay packs in many health-food stores. The prepared packs are sometimes even premixed with herbs and can be conveniently stored in the freezer and then put in the microwave or a pot of boiling water for a few minutes to make them ready for use.

To create a small clay pack yourself, mix 1 tablespoon of clay with several arthritis-fighting herbs (see Chapter 4 for the best herbs to use for arthritis) and mix until you have a thin paste. You might want to also add in a few drops of an herbal oil or olive oil, which will help the pack remain moist and make it easier to remove. Evenly spread the paste about a quarter of an inch thick onto a piece of cloth and apply it to the affected part of the body. You can purchase clay for this purpose at a good health-food store, from catalogs, or over the Internet.

Try a Cabbage Pack

For chronic cases of rheumatism and arthritis, alternating a clay pack with a pack made of pulped white cabbage can be very beneficial. A cabbage pack is very easy to make, and, since they have a gentle healing effect, its OK to place the leaves in direct contact with the skin, unlike with more stringent leaves.

Mash several white cabbage leaves into a paste and then heat them to a comfortable temperature in a steamer or microwave. Make sure that the paste is not too hot and then apply it directly to the affected area and wrap it with a piece of linen or other cloth.

Do not keep the pack on for longer than five minutes. A series of short applications with frequent breaks will do your joints more good than a single, long, uninterrupted application.

Herbal Packs for Relieving Pain

Some herbs are very effective when crushed and made into a pain-relieving paste by adding a little oil and water. Wrapped in a cloth and applied directly to the painful joints, these packs can be very efficient at driving off arthritic pain. Comfrey and horsetail are two pain-fighting superstars that are commonly recommended by herbalists.

Comfrey: Herbalists have long touted this plant as aiding in the healing of all types of bruises and even in speeding the healing of fractured bones. A comfrey pack may also be useful to those who suffer with varicose veins or gout. This soothing treatment has brought relief for many. To make a comfrey pack, take a couple of spoons of dried, crushed comfrey root and mix with enough hot water to make a paste. Add a few drops of cold-pressed olive oil and spread the mixture onto a cloth. Fold the cloth in half and apply to the sore area for five to 10 minutes.

Horsetail: Many herbalists recommend a pack made from horsetail to provide relief for arthritic pain. It is especially effective when allowed to remain on the affected area overnight. To make a horsetail pack, take several handfuls of the herb (available through most local health-food stores and from Internet sources) and steam it in a vegetable steamer until it is soft and hot. Wrap the steamed herb in a cloth, apply to the painful area, and fasten securely. You may want to wrap this pack with a second (larger) cloth to keep the moist heat from escaping.

Herbal Massages

A massage is a great way to help relieve the stiffness of sore muscles and aching joints. Whether you massage an aching joint or muscle yourself for a few minutes or go to a professional for a head-to-toe treatment, a massage will help promote relaxation, stretch the muscles, and improve circulation.

To increase the therapeutic value of your massage, you can use an oil infused with herbs reputed to have soothing, pain-fighting effects. Or try an ointment made with ingredients said to reduce inflammation or dampen arthritis-related pain. Following are several herbs that have been shown to be particularly effective as massage aids.

Marjoram Oil: One of the best massage oils for arthritic pain is marjoram oil. The warming effects of this herbal aid, combined with the gentle rubbing action of a massage, helps to relieve pain in aching joints and relax stiff muscles. Massage the oil gently into the affected area whenever relief is needed.

Directions for making marjoram oil: Use a spoon or a rolling pin to lightly crush enough of the herb to fill a glass jar halfway full. Do not use a plastic container. Fill the jar the rest of the way with olive oil, cap tightly, and place the bottle in a warm location. Allow the mixture to sit for three weeks. After three weeks, strain the herb-soaked oil and use it as a massage aid.

Saint-John's-wort Oil: Saint-John's-wort has traditionally been used as a natural treatment for pulled muscles and sprains. The herb has also shown promise as a treatment for the muscle-and-joint aches that accompany arthritis, helping to ease pain and stiffness.

Directions for making Saint-John's-wort Oil: Fill a glass jar about three-fourths of the way full with Saint-John's-wort (available through local health-food stores). Then fill the rest of the jar with cold-pressed olive oil. Cap tightly and place in a warm location for approximately three to four weeks. You will know when the mixture is ready to strain because it turns red. When the oil is ready, strain it and use it as a massage aid. Saint-John's-wort oil keeps its potency for up to two years as long as it is stored away from direct light.

Stinging Nettle: I have already mentioned that the Stinging Nettle herb is a useful arthritis treatment. Interestingly, the tea has been found to be quite an effective massage aid as well. Simply brew the tea as you would brew a cup of it to drink and allow it to cool to a tepid temperature. Apply the tea to painful areas and massage gently.

Shark Cartilage Cream

Recently, shark cartilage, a proven therapy for treating arthritis, has made an exciting new advance. Typically, the cartilage is administered orally in a powdered form. However, it appears that shark cartilage can also be absorbed directly through the skin. The obvious advantage to taking shark cartilage topically is that it can be delivered directly to the desired location with all of its constituents intact and with a minimum of fuss.

Scientists theorize that shark cartilage applied topically feeds joints a steady *meal* of cartilage-building nutrients so that the tissue breakdown is halted and new tissue can grow. Most commercial shark-cartilage creams combine shark cartilage with the highly effective counterirritant capsaicin. (See the next page for more information on capsaicin.) You should apply the cream directly to painful or swollen joints. Shark-cartilage creams can be found in local health-food stores and through the Internet.

Capsaicin

Capsaicin is a natural substance derived from cayenne pepper. It is what gives the peppers their hot spicy taste. This substance has been found to be an effective pain reliever. It works by lowering or depleting the chemical messenger in nerve cells (called decapeptide substance P) that transmits pain signals.

Capsaicin has been shown in clinical trials to ease a number of different kinds of pain, including postsurgical pain, neuralgic pain, osteoarthritic pain, and pain from rheumatoid arthritis. In one 16-week trial performed by the American Society of Clinical Oncology, capsaicin cream outperformed a placebo cream by a full 43%, with 60% of the trial participants being cured of their neuralgic pain during the 16-week period.

You should use capsaicin creams with caution, because some people are hypersensitive to the creams or to hot peppers in general and may experience a negative reaction. You should never use a cream on or near any areas of broken skin or near the eyes or mouth. Try to use gloves when applying the cream. If it is impossible to use gloves, be sure to wash your hands with soap and water after applying the cream—to avoid accidentally getting it in your eyes or on other sensitive areas. Use a small amount of the cream and rub it into the affected area completely, so that there is little to no cream left on the skin surface.

First-time users of the cream will normally experience a warm stinging or mild burning sensation, which often disappears after the first couple of days of use. You must continue to use the cream on a regular basis as directed by your doctor or in the instructions on the product in order for it to work and continue working. In the case of arthritic pain, it usually takes a week to two weeks of use to provide pain relief.

Topical creams containing capsaicin are available for purchase at your local health or natural-food store, through mail-order catalogs, or over the Internet. There are also joint-support creams available now that contain capsaicin in combination with other joint-supporting nutrients, including shark cartilage, glucosamine, and chondroitin.

Stimulating Circulation

As is the case with many ailments, arthritis and rheumatism are aggravated by, if not partially caused by, poor circulation. Stimulating your circulatory system, therefore, can greatly aid your arthritic condition.

The easiest way to stimulate circulation is by simply alternating hot and cold water when you take a shower and vigorously rubbing the skin with a washcloth or bath brush once or twice a day.

Similarly, a twice-weekly bath with Epsom salts, though an old-fashioned treatment, can be highly effective. Epsom salts' high mineral content (primarily magnesium sulphate) helps to soothe aching muscles and joints. Also consider stimulating circulation by massaging your painful joints with baking powder while they are submerged in the warm water.

Putting the Freeze on Arthritis

An excellent way to relieve your body of arthritic pain is through ice therapy. This is a simple, but effective, form of treatment and can be carried out with just an ordinary ice pack or two basins of water.

Fill an ice pack with up to 10 ice cubes and apply it below or above the joint that hurts. Do not put it directly on the joint. Wrap a towel around the pack and let it sit snugly for about 30 minutes. You will, of course, initially feel the cold from the ice pack, but this sensation soon changes to a warming one and eventually turns into a slightly numb feeling. The end result is often a reduction in pain and swelling and welcome relief for several hours. You may repeat this treatment several times throughout the day as needed for pain relief.

If your hands or feet are afflicted with arthritis, a contrast bath is an excellent remedy. You will need two basins. Fill the first with ice water and the other with water that is comfortably hot. Do not make the water so hot that you cannot comfortably place your hands or feet into it.

Soak the affected area in the hot water for about 10 minutes. Then place your sore joints into the cold water for no longer than one minute. Continue this pattern for 30 minutes. Not only will you notice that your pain has eased, but you will discover that your fingers or toes are more mobile. For maximum benefit, you should end the session with one minute in a cold bath.

> **T I P**
>
> While most forms of bodywork (such as using ice-packs, taking warm footbaths, or massage) have no negative side effects for the majority of people, those with diabetes, Reynaud's Syndrome, or collagen or blood conditions should use hydrotherapy and ice therapy only under a physician's supervision.

Stimulating Footbaths

A warm electric footbath can at best improve the circulation of blood throughout the body and at least alleviate the pain and stiffness associated with arthritis.

For an extra healing boost, you can add herbal blends to your footbath. A stimulating footbath gradually raises the temperature of the body. The benefits begin in the feet by first expanding the tiny capillaries in the soles. As the temperature slowly rises, the deep-seated, larger arterioles and the large blood vessels of the feet expand. In a relatively short period of time, all the blood vessels of the feet are expanded as far as possible and the therapeutic effects of the warming and any herbs that are used are felt throughout the body.

The footbath can be used to soak not only your feet but also—if it is placed on a raised surface—your hands and elbows as well. Electric footbaths can be found in most large retail stores that sell household and bath supplies.

Paraffin Baths

Paraffin baths work very effectively for soothing chronic joint pain and inflammation. You simply use the bath unit to heat the paraffin wax to a comfortable temperature that is normally around 120 degrees to 130 degrees Fahrenheit. Next, you dip the affected hand, foot, or elbow into the wax for about 15 minutes. After 15 minutes, it is easy to remove the wax from your skin.

Users report that the penetrating heat provides pain relief and is very relaxing.

One recent study by the Institute of Population Health concluded that paraffin baths are effective and have beneficial short-term effects on arthritic conditions.

Paraffin baths are nothing new. In fact, studies evaluating their effectiveness for pain relief can be found in the literature dating back to at least the early 1970s. Until recently, however, paraffin treatments had to be confined to a physical therapist's office or a doctor's office. Now, affordable and safe portable units are available in most drug stores, in small-appliance stores, and over the Internet. Some insurance companies will even pay for, or offset the cost of, a portable paraffin bath when your doctor recommends it.

Chiropractic

A 1999 study published in the *Annals of Internal Medicine* revealed that 63% of arthritis and fibromyalgia patients who sought care from a rheumatologist also sought care from a complementary- and alternative-care (CAM) practitioner. Chiropractic care was at the top of the list for the kinds of CAM care patients sought.

Chiropractic care is based on evaluating the spine to determine if any part of it is malfunctioning or causing abnormal body movements. When that's the case, these malfunctions, called *subluxations*, are thought to contribute to the overall stress on the nervous system and therefore compromise the health and well-being of the patient. The chiropractor administers spinal adjustments that are designed to diminish or eliminate stress on the nerves, thereby promoting normal function, range of motion, and healing. Chiropractors employ a variety of pain-reduction tools, including hot or cold packs, ultrasound treatments, and mild electrical stimulation to sore areas.

As chiropractic care is increasingly accepted by the medical mainstream, some insurance companies will now cover such treatment. Check with your insurance carrier to see if it will cover or offset the cost of chiropractic treatment. The best way to find a good chiropractor is to ask family members and friends for a recommendation. You can also contact the National Center for Complimentary and Alternative Medicine (NCCAM). Information on getting in touch with the NCCAM can be found in Appendix I of this book.

Acupuncture

The theory behind acupuncture is that illness is caused by imbalances and energy blocks in the body. The acupuncturist stimulates the release of energy along the main energy lines, or *meridians*, in the body, allowing and stimulating the body to heal. Thin needles, heat, and occasionally magnets are used in the practice of acupuncture.

Even though acupuncture has been successfully practiced in China for more than 2,000 years, acceptance in the West has been an uphill climb. One of the main difficulties is that Western science is not yet able to confirm and measure the energy lines upon which acupuncture is based. Therefore, its success is considered primarily theoretical and anecdotal—being passed along by word-of-mouth.

Nevertheless, so many people, including osteoarthritis and fibromyalgia patients, have done so well with acupuncture that the U.S. National Institutes of Health has launched a massive study in order to draw conclusions and recommendations regarding its effectiveness. A number of studies over the years have shown it to be an effective treatment for a variety of painful conditions caused by cancer, back injuries, and arthritis. Scientists at the University of Exeter conducted an analysis of 12 recent clinical trials involving acupuncture. That study, the results of which were published in the April 2002 issue of the highly regarded medical journal *Der Schmerz*, concluded that the collected data showed acupuncture to be superior to other control interventions. It turns out that the odds of seeing an improvement in pain control were better when acupuncture was used than when any of the other methods studied in the 12 trials was employed.

Increasing numbers of doctors, especially rheumatologists who specialize in arthritis, are beginning to accept acupuncture as a good adjunct therapy for the treatment of arthritic pain. To find an experienced acupuncturist, ask your doctor or local hospital for a recommendation. You can also contact the National Certification Commission for Acupuncture and Oriental Medicine (NCCAOM). Contact information for the organization can be found in Appendix I at the back of this book.

Acupressure

Acupressure has its foundation in acupuncture, but there is a major difference; instead of using needles, the acupressurist uses touch. By pressing on specific energy points and sore spots, the acupressurist stimulates the release of energy to affected areas— boosting circulation and bringing about pain relief. *Shiatsu*, roughly translated from the Chinese as *finger pressure*, is a slightly more vigorous method of acupressure. Your doctor or local health spa can probably refer you to a good acupressurist. The National Certification Commission for Acupuncture and Oriental Medicine (NCCAOM) has begun a certification program for Oriental bodywork therapy, which includes the practice of acupressure. You may contact that organization for more information, (Check Appendix I at the back of this book.) Information on acupressure can also be obtained from the Acupressure Institute. (Again, check Appendix I for contact information.)

EPILOGUE

Good health is not something that just happens to you. It takes discipline, hard work, and determination. But the rewards are enormous.

That is why more of us are taking direct control of our bodies and learning more about how we can claim good health as our own and how we can maintain it. We all deserve to live our lives to the fullest, pain-free and free of worry. This book is intended as a tool to get you started on the road to health. It is just one resource to use on your journey.

Throughout this volume, I have explained how various supplements or products may make your quest for robust health easier. We have covered a lot of ground here. But there is no need to feel overwhelmed. Simply take your journey toward a pain-free life one step at a time. Discuss different alternative-treatment options with your doctor or other medical practitioner. Choose some treatments or therapies that appeal to you and give them a try. And don't be discouraged if something does not seem to work as well for you as it has for some; not every treatment or solution works for everyone. If you'll just be patient and persistent, you'll find that you have much more control over your situation than you ever thought possible.

Although I have discussed a large variety of the latest options and long-term proven techniques, there is not, of course, room for everything on the horizon. New discoveries and breakthroughs are being made everyday. It is entirely possible that by the time you are reading this book a new treatment or therapy will have been proven to be a success. So use this book as it was intended: as a resource and starting point to answer your questions about arthritis. Whenever you have a question regarding arthritis or your treatment options, consult this book first; you are bound to find the answer you are seeking.

We sincerely hope that *HOW TO FIGHT ARTHRITIS & WIN* helps you to lead a healthier, happier, and more robust life. Please feel free to share your experiences, questions, and comments with us. May good health be yours!

Resources for Learning More About Arthritis and Natural Healing Methods

Your local library will have listings of organizations, support groups, and alternative-health-care resources for learning more about joint support and living with arthritis. Libraries also provide access to the Internet for people who don't have computers at home.

By using Internet search engines, such as yahoo.com and google.com, you will be able to learn about and access numerous Internet sites that provide additional information and personal testimonials on arthritis and natural healing (as well as chat rooms, message boards, and on-line support groups).

Listed on the next few pages are some selected resources to get you started.

ACUPRESSURE INSTITUTE

1533 Shattuck Ave.
Berkeley, CA 94709
Phone: (510) 845-1059

The Acupressure Institute provides training in various styles of acupressure and offers the public general information as well as a mail-order catalog of publications.

ARTHRITIS FOUNDATION

P.O. Box 7669
Atlanta, GA 30357-0669
Phone: (800) 283-7800
website: www.arthritis.org
e-mail: help@arthritis.org

There are many local chapters of the Arthritis Foundation in all 50 states and Washington, D.C. Call, write, or go on-line to find the chapter nearest you. The Arthritis Foundation also provides valuable booklets and other materials on living with arthritis.

HEALTH SCIENCES INSTITUTE

819 N. Charles St.
Baltimore, MD 21201
Phone: (800) 981-7157
website: www.hsibaltimore.com
e-mail: hsiresearch@agora-inc.com

The Health Sciences Institute (HSI) is a group made up of researchers, scientists, and health practitioners worldwide, joined together in a research-driven medical network. It offers a monthly newsletter, daily free e-Alerts, and a variety of information on cutting-edge therapies, cures, and treatments.

NATIONAL CENTER FOR COMPLEMENTARY AND ALTERNATIVE MEDICINE (NCCAM)

P.O. Box 7923
Gaithersburg, MD 20898
Phone: (888) 644-6226 (toll-free)
International: (301) 519-3153
TTY: (86) 464-3615 (toll-free)
FAX: (866) 464-3616 (toll-free)
website: nccam.nih.gov
e-mail: info@nccam.nih.gov

The NCCAM is an organization dedicated to exploring complementary and alternative healing practices in the context of rigorous science, training CAM researchers, and disseminating authoritative information to the public and professionals.

NATIONAL CERTIFICATION COMMISSION FOR ACUPUNCTURE AND ORIENTAL MEDICINE (NCCAOM)

11 Canal Center Plaza, Suite 300
Alexandria, VA 22314
Phone: (703) 548-9004
Fax: (703) 548-9079
website: www.NCCAOM.org
e-mail: info@nccaom.org

The NCCAOM is a nonprofit organization that has as its mission to promote nationally recognized standards of competency and safety in acupuncture and Oriental medicine for the purpose of protecting the public.

NATIONAL INSTITUTE OF ARTHRITIS AND
MUSCULOSKELETAL AND SKIN DISEASES (NIAMS)
INFORMATION CLEARINGHOUSE

1 AMS Circle
Bethesda, MD 20892-3675
Phone: (877) 226-4267 (toll-free)
TTY: (301) 565-2966
website: www.niams.nih.gov
e-mail: niamsinfo@mail.nih.gov

The NIAMS is currently conducting large-scale clinical trials on glucosamine and chondroitin for the treatment of arthritis. It also provides a number of informative booklets and pamphlets on arthritic conditions and arthritis research.

NORTHSTAR NUTRITIONALS

P.O. Box 925
Frederick, MD 21705
Phone: (800) 311-1950 (and ask for code M650C209)
website: www.northstarnutritionals.com

NorthStar Nutritionals is the manufacturer of high-quality nutritional products including their exclusive joint-support formula that combines MSM with 10 other natural pain-fighting and joint-supporting ingredients.

W E B   R E S O U R C E S

www.arthritisinsight.com

This informative Web resource is maintained by and for people with arthritis and includes message boards, chat rooms, and other useful links.

Arthritis Insight
P.O. Box 441571
Indianapolis IN 46244
e-mail: info@arthritisinsight.com

http://home.gci.net/~cushman4/oa-gcs.htm

This website is an information resource focused on helping individuals with OA make informed decisions about glucosamine/chondroitin sulphate and other supplements. It is privately maintained and does not sell products or accept advertising.

www.alternatives4arthritis.com

Alternatives 4 Arthritis provides valuable information about mind-body healing methods, such as yoga and meditation, for arthritis patients. The site is privately maintained by Ellen Gordon, a writer and researcher who has lived with rheumatoid arthritis for 20 years.

www.holisticonline.com

Holisticonline provides comprehensive information about conventional, alternative, integrative, and mind-body medicine for healing common ailments and conditions.

www.egregore.com

This website is called Medicinal Herbs Online. It serves as an information clearinghouse for medicinal herbs, including links for purchasing herbal products on-line.

www.arthritissupport.com

ArthritisSupport.com is the Pro Health, Inc. website that focuses on three primary objectives: reporting the latest news in arthritis treatment and research, making quality nutritional supplements available directly from the manufacturers at low prices, and supporting arthritis research by donating profits on remedy purchases.

www.drtheo.com

This is the official website for Dr. Jason Theodosakis, author of *The Arthritis Cure* and other books about glucosamine, chondroitin, and health care. The information is focused on healing methods for osteoarthritis and general joint support.

www.northstarnutritionals.com

NorthStar Nutritionals is a manufacturer of high-quality nutritional products, including Flexanol designed to maintain normal joint functioning with natural ingredients.

LABS THAT CONDUCT MYCOPLASMA TESTING

INSTITUTE FOR MOLECULAR MEDICINE

15162 Triton Lane
Hunting Beach, CA 92649-1041
Phone: (714) 903-2900

IMMUNOSCIENCES LABORATORY

8730 Wilshire Blvd., Suite 305
Beverly Hills, CA 90211
Phone: (800) 950-4686 or (310) 657-1077

• APPENDIX II •

Selected Bibliography

Airola, Paavo, N.D., Ph. D., *How to Get Well*, Health Plus Publishers, Phoenix, Arizona, 1974

Alexander, Dale, *Arthritis and Common Sense*, Simon and Schuster, New York, 1981

Arthritis and Nutrition, Nutritional Education Association, Inc., Houston, Texas, 1983

Christensen, Alice, *The American Yoga Association's Easy Does It Yoga: The Safe and Gentle Way to Health and Well-Being*, Simon and Schuster, New York, 1999

Cooper, Jean, *The Food Pharmacy*, Bantam Books, New York, 1988

Eisenstein, Phyllis, Ph.D., *Overcoming the Pain of Inflammatory Arthritis*, Avery Publishing Group, Garden City Park, New York, 1997

Fischer, William L., *How to Fight Cancer & Win*, Agora Health Books, Baltimore, Maryland, 2000

Fischer, William L., *Miracle Healing Through Nature's Pharmacy*, Fischer Publishing Co., Canfield, Ohio, 1986

Fredericks, Carlton, Ph.D., *Arthritis: Don't Learn to Live With It,* Grosset and Dunlap, New York, 1981

Heinerman, John, *Heinerman's Encyclopedia of Fruits, Vegetables, and Herbs,* Parker Publishing Co., New York, 1988

Hou, FaXiang, Master, *Unleashing the Power of Food: Recipes to Heal By,* Agora Health Books, Baltimore, 2001

Integrative Medicine Access, *Professional Reference to Conditions, Herbs, and Supplements,* Integrative Medicine Communications, Newton, Massachusetts, 2000

Jarvis, D.C., M.D., *Arthritis and Folk Medicine,* Pan Books, London, 1972

Jensen, Bernard, Ph.D., *Arthritis, Rheumatism, and Osteoporosis,* Dr. Bernard Jensen, Publisher, Escondido, California, 1986

Jensen, Bernard, Ph.D., *Nature Has a Remedy,* Dr. Bernard Jensen, Publisher, Escondido, California, 1984

Kalyn, Wayne, Editor, *The Healing Power of Vitamins, Minerals, and Herbs,* Reader's Digest Association, Inc., Pleasantville, New York, 1999

Kandel, Joseph, M.D. and David Sudderth, M.D., *The Anti-Arthritis Diet,* Prima Health, Rocklin, CA, 1998

Keough, Carol, *Natural Relief for Arthritis,* Rodale Press, Emmaus, Pennsylvania, 1983

Lee, R.Ph., Ph.D., *The Book of Raw Fruit and Vegetable Juices and Drinks,* Keats Publishing, Inc., New Canaan, Connecticut, 1982

Long, Ph.D., and Ruth Yale, *A Basic Diet Plan and Use of Food Supplements*, Nutrition Education Association, Inc., Houston, 1983

McDougall, John A., M.D., *McDougall's Medicine: A Challenging Second Opinion*, New Century Publishers, Inc., Piscataway, New Jersey, 1985

Mervyn, Leonard, Ph.D., *Thorsons' Complete Guide To Vitamins and Minerals*, Thorsons Publishers, Inc., Rochester, Vermont, 1987

Miller, Lucinda G., PharmD, BCPS and Wallace J. Murray, Ph.D., *Herbal Medicinals: A Clinician's Guide*, Pharmaceutical Products Press, Binghamton, New York, 1998

Milner, Martin, N.D., Medical Editor, *Underground Cures: The Most Urgent Health Secrets III Edition*, Agora Health Books, Baltimore, Maryland, 2001

Monro, Robin, Dr., Dr. R. Nagarathna, and Dr. H.R. Nagendra, *Yoga for Common Ailments*, Simon & Schuster Inc., New York, 1990

Rooney, Theodore W., M.D., and Patty Ryan Rooney, *The Arthritis Handbook*, Ballentine Books, New York, 1985

Scala, James, M.D., *The Arthritis Relief Diet*, Penguin Books, New York, 1987

Trattler, Ross, M.D., *Better Health Through Natural Healing*, McGraw-Hill Book Co., New York, 1988

Walker, N.W., *Raw Vegetable Juices*, The Berkeley Publishing Group, New York, 1984

INDEX

boldface indicates boxed text   underscore indicates chart

italic indicates diagram

A

Achilles tendon, and bursitis, 5

Acupressure, 134

Acupuncture, 105, 133–134

Adaptive immunity, 11

Adler, Patricia, 121

Advil, 29

Age
  and ankylosing spondylitis, 21
  and caloric intake, 36–37
  and osteoarthritis, 1–2, *2*
  and rheumatoid arthritis, 10

American College of Rheumatology, 23

American Journal of Clinical Dermatology, 79

American Society of Clinical Oncology, 128

Ankylosing spondylitis, 20–21, 23–24

Annals of Internal Medicine, 132

Annals of Rheumatic Diseases, 44

Antibiotics, 13

Antidepressants, natural, 88

Antioxidants, 66

Apple-cider vinegar and honey, 78–80

Aquatic exercises, 110–114

Archives of Internal Medicine, 29

Arthritis Foundation, 1, 2, 18, 110–111

Aseptic meningitis, 29

Aspirin, 29, 68, 82

Attitude and arthritis, 31, 32

Autoimmune disease, 11, 87

Ayurvedic herbs, 102–104

B

Bacteria and rheumatoid arthritis, 12–14

Bathtub exercises, 112–114

Bee products, 76–77

Bioflavonoids, 68–71

Bipolar disorder, 89

Black-current oil, 91–92

Bodywork
acupressure, 134
acupuncture, 103–104, 105, 133–134
chiropractic, 132

Bones
and boron, 75
and calcium, 71–73
and joint capsules, 4–5
and osteophytes, 5
and vitamin D, 66–67

Borage oil, 91–92

Boron, 74–76

Boswellia, 103–104

Bottle brush, 98

Bovine spongiform encephalopathy (BSE), 84–85

Breathing, controlled deep, 34, 114–115

British Journal of Nutrition, 45

Burks, Thomas, 61

Bursae, 4

Bursitis, 4–5

C

Cabbage packs, 124–125

Caffeine, 62–63, 72, 95

Calcium, 45–46, 52, 71–73, 79, 94

Cancer, 92–94, 95

Capsaicin, 60–62, 128–129

Carbohydrates, refined, 36

Carbonated soft drinks, 46

Carpal tunnel syndrome, 24–25

Carrots, 57–58

Cartilage, 4–5, 21, 36, 52

Celebrex, 28, 29

Center for Special Immunology, 13

Cervical spondylosis, 8

Childers, Dr. Norman F., 43

Children, and juvenile rheumatoid arthritis, 18

Chili peppers, 60–62

Chiropractic, 132

Chondroitin, 83–86, 93, 94

Chronic Fatigue Syndrome and Fibromyalgia Clinic, 13

Chronic pattern of rheumatoid arthritis, 10

Circulation, stimulating, 129

Citric acid allergies, 53, 54

Clay packs, 123–124

Cleansing diets, 38–39

Club moss, 97

Coburn, James, 86–87

Cod-liver oil, 51–54

Cold-water ocean fish, 54–55

Colitis, 23–24

Collagen, 94

Colloidal silver, 13–14

Comfrey, 125

Complementary medicine, 30, 132

Copper, 80

Cox-2 inhibitors, 28–29

Crepitant sounds, 7

Crohn's disease, 23

Curcumin, 104

D

Dandelion, 99–100

Devil's claw, 101–102

Diabetes, 86

Diet
    and age, 36–37
    and arthritis management plans,
    31, 32

calcium in the, 45–46, 52, 71–73

carrots in the, 57–58

chili peppers in the, 60–62

and citric acid allergies, 53, 54

cleansing, 38–39

digestive enzymes in the, 41–42

disease promoting, 36

and dryness in the body, 48, 53

essential fatty acids (EFAs) in the,
    47–55

flaxseed (linseed) oil in the, 49–51

fruits and vegetables as main com-
    ponents of, 55–57

and gout, 22, 57, 97

green tea in the, 62–63, 71, 94–95

healing power of, 35–36

hidden food sensitivities and,
    39–40, 43–44

and juicing, 58

magnesium in the, 46

and metabolism, 36–37, 49–50

nightshades in the, 43–44

permanent, health-promoting,
    42–43

phosphorus in the, 45–46

and preparing fresh vegetables,
    58–59

prostaglandins in the, 49–50

refined carbohydrates in the, 36

royal jelly in the, 76–77

and tobacco, 43, 44

Digestive enzymes, 41–42

Dopamine, 88

Dry skin, 48, 53

Dutch rushes, 98

E

Eggplant, 43–44

Eicosapentaenoic acid (EPA), 54–55

Elbows, and bursitis, 5

Embrel, 30

Emotions and arthritis, 14–18

Epsom salts, 129

Essential fatty acids (EFAs), 47–55

Evening-primrose oil, 91–92

Exercise
and aging, 107–108
aquatic, 110–114
and arthritis management plans, 31
bathtub, 112–114
and deep breathing, 34, 114–115
Pilates, 119–120
and relaxation, 17–18, 115–116
and stress, 17
stretching, 116–118
and symptoms of osteoarthritis, 6
tai chi, 120–121
walking as, 109–110
yoga, 17, 118–119

F

Feet
and bursitis, 5
and gout, 22

Felson, Dr. David T., 37

Feverfew, 100–101

Fibromyalgia, 23, 132

Financial costs of arthritis, 1

Finger swing exercises, 113

First National Health and Nutrition Examination Survey, 37

Fish, cold-water ocean, 54–55

FitzGerald, Dr. Garret A., 29

Flavonoids, 95

Flaxseed (linseed) oil, 49–51, 92

Folic acid, 80–81, 88

Food and Drug Administration (FDA), 29

Food sensitivities, hidden, 39–40, 43–44

Foot stretches, 113–114

Foot synchronization, 113

Footbaths, 130–131

Framingham Heart Study, 37

Free radicals, 66, 95

Fruits, 55–57, 68–71

Fusing, 21

G

Gallic acid, 62

Gamma-linoleic acid (GLA), 91–92

Gelling, 5

Gender
and arthritis, 11–12, 19, 21
and calcium, 72
and gout, 23

Genetics and arthritis, 21

Gesundheitswesen, 70

Ginger, 95–96

Glucosamine, 83–86, 94

Gokshura, **103**

Gout, 22–23, 57, 97, 99

Granulomatous colitis, 23

Green tea, 62–63, 71, 94–95

Guduchi, **103**

Guggul, **103**

H

Hands and wrists
  and carpal tunnel syndrome, 24–25
  and osteoarthritis, 6–7
  and rheumatoid arthritis, 8–9
Head and neck
  and osteoarthritis, 7–8
  and rheumatoid arthritis, 9
  stretches, 118
Health Sciences Institute, 12
Heart disease, 28–29, 54, 95, 102, 109
Heberden's nodes, 5
Herbal remedies
  Ayurvedic, 102–104
  boswellia, 103–104
  capsaicin, 60–62, 128–129
  club moss, 97
  comfrey, 125
  dandelion, 99–100
  devil's claw, 101–102
  feverfew, 100–101
  gamma-linoleic acid (GLA), 91–92
  ginger, 95–96
  glucosamine and chondroitin, 83–86, 93–94
  green tea, 62–63, 71, 94–95
  horsetail, 97–98, 125
  lyprinol, 89–91
  marjoram oil, 126
  for massages, 126–127
    methyl sulfonyl methane (MSM), 86–88
    s-adenosylmethionine (SAMe), 88–89
    Saint-John's-wort oil, 126–127
    shark cartilage, 92–94, 127
    stinging nettle, 99, 127
    topical, 125–131
    Traditional Chinese Medicine (TCM), 104–105
    yarrow, 98
Hip rotators, 117–118
Hippocrates, 78
Holistic and natural healing, 28
Horseradish tree, **103**
Horsetail, 97–98, 125
How to Fight Cancer & Win, 47–48
How to Fight Heart Disease & Win, 55
Hypertension, 22
Hypoglycemia, 62

I

Ibuprofen, 29, 82
Ice therapy, 129–130
Immune malfunction and rheumatoid arthritis, 11–12
  and food sensitivities, 40, 41
  and green tea, 95
Indian Frankincense, 103–104
Indian madder, **103**
Inflammatory bowel diseases, 23–24
Insulin resistance, 86

J

Joints
    and ankylosing spondylitis, 20–21
    and bursitis, 4–5
    and cartilage, 4–5
    and crepitant sounds, 7
    effects of obesity on, 36–37
    and gelling, 5
    and gout, 22
    healthy, 4
    with osteoarthritis, **6**
    and osteophytes, 5
    with rheumatoid arthritis, **9**
    and synovial membranes, 5

Journal of Nutrition, 62

Journal of the American Medical Association (JAMA), 28, 85

Juicing, 58

Juvenile rheumatoid arthritis, 18

K

Kadler, Nancy, 112

Kidney failure, 29

Knees
    and bursitis, 5
    stretching, 117
    and swimming, 111
    and ulcerative-colitis, 23–24

L

Lancet, 29, 45, 85

Licorice, **103**

Life charts, 15, **16**

Lind, Dr. James, 68

Lyprinol, 89–91

M

Mad cow disease, 84–85

Magnesium, 46, 73, 75

Management plans, arthritis. *see also* Treatments
    basic components of, 32
    complementary healing as part of, 30
    controlled deep breathing in, 34, 114–115
    and holistic and natural healing defined, 28
    pharmaceutical medicines in, 30, 82
    visualization and relaxation in, 32, 33–34, 114–116

Manganese, 81

Marjoram oil, 126

Massages, herbal, 126–127

Mayo clinic, 20

Meat consumption and arthritis, 42, 44–46

Media coverage of arthritis, 1

Meditation, 32, 33–34

Meningitis, 29

Meridians, 133

Metabolism, 36–37, 49–50

Methyl sulfonyl methane (MSM), 86–88

Milner, Dr. Martin, 93

Mind, healing power of the, 32, 33–34

Minerals, 45–46, 52, 71–76, 80–82, 94

Monocyclic pattern of rheumatoid arthritis, 10

Motrin, 29

Multiple sclerosis, 30

Muscles
    and healthy joints, 4
    weakness in, 8

Musk mallow, **103**

Mycoplasmas, 12–14

N

National Academy of Sciences, 62, 95

National Center for Complimentary and Alternative Medicine (NCCAM), 132

National Certification Commission for Acupuncture and Oriental Medicine (NCCAOM), 134

National Institute of Arthritis and Musculoskeletal and Skin Diseases (NIAMS), 2

National Institutes of Health, 83, 120, 133

New England Journal of Medicine, 29

New Zealand green-lipped mussels, 89–91

Newnham, Dr. Rex E., 74–75

Nightshades, 43–44

Nodules, skin, 9

Nonsteroidal anti-inflammatory drugs, 29, 84, 88

Nutritional supplements
    apple-cider vinegar and honey as, 78–80
    herbal, 83–105
    mineral, 45–46, 52, 71–76, 80–82, 88
    propolis, 77–78
    royal jelly, 76–77
    shark cartilage, 92–94
    vitamin, 66–71

O

Obesity, 22, 36–38, 95

Osteoarthritis
    and age, 1–2
    areas of the body affected by, **2**
    and calcium, 71–73
    and cartilage, 4–5
    and diet, 37–38
    in the hand and wrist, 6–7
    in the neck, 7–8
    prevalence of, 1, 2
    primary, 3
    secondary, 3
    and shark cartilage, 92–94
    symptoms of, 2, 6–8
    types of, 3
    and vitamin D, 66–67

Osteophytes, 5

Oxygen supplements, 14

P

Pain

and acupuncture, 103–104, 105, 133–134
and bioflavonoids, 70
and capsaicin, 60–62
and devil's claw, 101–102
and exercise, 114
and feverfew, 100–101
and food sensitivities, 39–40
and ginger, 95–96
and glucosamine and chondroitin, 84
and herbal packs, 125
management through visualization and meditation, 32, 33–34
and methyl sulfonyl methane (MSM), 87
relieving properties of carrots, 57–58
and royal jelly, 76–77
as symptom of arthritis, 6–8, 9, 19, 21, 23
tolerance levels, 31
and vitamin B5, 71
and vitamin E, 66
and zinc, 73–74
Pantothenic acid, 71, 78
Paraffin baths, 131–132
Parkinson's disease, 89
Parthenolide, 100–101
Peppers, 43–44
Peripheral arthritis, 24
Pewterwort, 98
Pharmaceutical medications, 28–30, 72, 82
Phosphorus, 45–46, 72, 75, 79, 94

Pilates exercises, 119–120
Polycyclic pattern of rheumatoid arthritis, 10
Potatoes, 43–44
Prevalence
    of osteoarthritis, 1, 2
    of rheumatoid arthritis, 1
Primary osteoarthritis, 3
Progressive relaxation, 33–34, 115–116
Propolis, 77–78
Prostaglandins, 49–50, 55, 100
Psoriatic arthritis, 19–20

R

Relaxation, 17–18, 114–116
Remicade, 30
Reynaud's syndrome, 34, 92
Rheumatic Diseases Clinics of North America, **105**
Rheumatism, 97, 99
Rheumatoid arthritis
    and age, 10
    and ankylosing spondylitis, 20–21
    areas of the body affected by, 8
    and bacteria, 12–14
    causes of, 10–15
    and diet, 59–60
    and exercise, 17
    and fibromyalgia, 23
    genetic causes of, 11–12
    and gout, 22–23
    and immune malfunction, 11–12

joint affected by, **9**
juvenile, 18
mortality from, 9
and mycoplasmas, 12–14
patterns of, 10
prevalence of, 1, 8
and psoriatic arthritis, 19–20
and relaxation, 17–18
and routines, 17–18
and shark cartilage, 93
and skin nodules, 9
and stress, 14–18
symptoms of, 8–9
and systemic lupus erythematosus, 18–19
and tobacco use, 44
and viruses, 12
and vitamin D, 66

Rose hips, 70

Routines and stress, 17–18

Royal jelly, 76–77

S

S-adenosylmethionine (SAMe),
88–89

Sacroiliac, 21

Saint-John's-wort oil, 126–127

Scurvy, 68–69

Seated stretch, 117

Secondary osteoarthritis, 3

See, Dr. Darryl, 13

Selenium, 14, 81–82

Shark cartilage, 92–94
cream, 127

Shave grass, 98

Shiatsu, 134

Shoulders, and bursitis, 4

Silicon, 97

Sjogren's syndrome, 92

Skin nodules, 9

Smoking, 43, 44

Solanine, 43

Spine
and ankylosing spondylitis,
20–21
and chiropractic, 132
and inflammatory bowel diseases, 24
and rheumatoid arthritis, 8–9

Standing stretch, 117

Statistics, arthritis, 1

Steroids, 72

Stinging nettle, 99, 127

Stress
and arthritis, 14–18, 33–34
walking to relieve, 110

Stretching exercises, 116–118

Subluxations, 132

Sulfur, 87

Support groups, 31

Swedish Bitters, 99

Swelling around joints, 7, 73–74, 90

Symptoms
of drying out, 48
of gout, 22
of osteoarthritis, 2, 6–8

positive and negative efffects on, 27
of psoriatic arthritis, 19–20
of rheumatoid arthritis, 8–9
of systemic lupus erythematosus, 18–19

Synovial fluid and membranes, 4, 5, 8, 21, 38

Systemic lupus erythematosus, 18–19, 87

Szent-Gyorgyi, Dr. Albert, 69

T

Tai chi, 120–121

Tenderness around joints, 7

Tendons, 4

Tenosynovitis, 24–25

Thumb cross exercises, 114

Thunder god vine, **105**

Tobacco, 43, 44

Toe hold exercises, 114

Tomatoes, 43–44

Topical remedies
cabbage pack, 124–125
capsaicin, 128–129
clay pack, 123–124
footbaths as, 130–131
herbal massage, 126–127
ice therapy, 129–130
paraffin baths as, 131–132
for relieving pain, 125
shark cartilage, 127
for stimulating circulation, 129

Traditional Chinese Medicine (TCM), 104–105

Trauma, and carpal tunnel syndrome, 24

Treatments. *see also* Management plans, arthritis
antiobiotc, 13
colloidal silver, 13–14
dangers of pharmaceutical medications for, 28–30, 72, 82
and life charts, 15, **16**
traditional, 27

Trigger foods, 39–40

Tuberculosis, 30

Tunder god vine, 105

Turmeric, 104

U

Ulcerative-colitis, 23–24

Ulcers, 29

Uric acid, 22, 57

V

Vaccinations, 11

Vegetables, 55–57, 58–59

Vinegar, 78–80

Vioxx, 28, 29, 82

Viruses and rheumatoid arthritis, 12

Visualization, 32, 33–34

Vitamins
B5, 71
B12, 88
C, 67–68

Vitamins, *continued*
    D, 66–67
    E, 66
    P, 68–71

W

Walking for exercise, 109–110
West, Dr. James R., 70
White blood cells, 13

Whitehouse, Dr. Michael, 90–91
Williams, Dr. Roger, 71

Y

Yarrow, 98
Yoga, 17, 118–119

Z

Zinc, 73–74

Don't miss these great books in the groundbreaking How to Fight series:

- *How to Fight Cancer & Win—*
  over 150,000 copies sold
- *How to Fight Prostate Cancer & Win*
- *How to Fight Arthritis & Win*
- *How to Fight Heart Disease & Win*

Dear Loyal Reader,

One of the best things you can do for your health is also one of the simplest; become an informed patient. It may seem almost too simple, but studies show that being more informed can actually lead to shortened hospital stays and less overall fatigue, disability, and health distress. It seems that the more we know about our health and the illnesses that threaten our well being, the better off we are.

We have made it our mission here at Agora Health Books to provide you with the most up-to-date and un-biased health information we can find; information that you can put into action. Only books that meet our most stringent standards are chosen to be included in our **How to Fight & Win** series. As a result you can trust that each book in this unique series is written in an even-handed and easy-to-understand manner, and is packed with actionable advice that you can begin to put to work for you right away.

These all-in-one source books are designed to give you the straight story on mainstream, complementary, and natural approaches to specific illnesses. Unlike some of the other biased books you might have run across in the past, each title in the **How to Fight & Win** series take a balanced and fair look at all the methods of preventing and treating an illness or disease.

You don't need to be a doctor to make decisions about your health. What you do need is to be able to see the bigger picture. With a complete understanding of the illnesses that threaten your well being, and the latest information on the best conventional, and alternative prevention and treatment options, you will finally be in the driver's seat and on the road to good health.

Don't wait any longer to take control and begin making educated health-care choices. Become an active participant in your own health-care decisions. Order your **How to Fight & Win** books now and experience what it is like to feel informed, empowered, and in total control of your health.

To your good health,

Alice E. Jacob

Alice E. Jacob, Managing Editor
Agora Health Books

Order Form

To order any of the books in the **How to Fight Series** simply check the title(s) of the book(s) you want, fill in the number of copies you wish to order, add in the appropriate amount of shipping and handling (see box below), and mail in this completed form.

❏ **How to Fight Cancer & Win** ___ copy/copies at **$19.95** ea. $_____
[680SFCBK]

❏ **How to Fight Prostate Cancer & Win** ___ copy/copies at **$19.95** ea. $_____
[680SBPRO]

❏ **How to Fight Arthritis & Win** ___ copy/copies at **$19.95** ea. $_____
[680SHFA]

❏ **How to Fight Heart Disease & Win** ___ copy/copies at **$19.95** ea. $_____
[680SFHD]

1-3 books add $5.00 shipping and handling	**SUBTOTAL**: $_____
4-9 books add $10.00 shipping and handling	**SHIPPING & HANDLING**: $_____
10+ books add $15.00 shipping and handling	(see S&H box for details)

TOTAL: $_____

Check method of payment: *(All orders processed in US dollars.)*

❏ My check is enclosed for $ _____ made payable to **Agora Health Books**.
  (Maryland residents add 5% sales tax)

❏ Please charge my: ❏ Visa ❏ MasterCard ❏ American Express ❏ Discover

Card #:_____ Expires:_____

Signature:_____

Ship to:

Name:_____

Address:_____

City:_____ State:_____ Zip:_____

Phone: (_____)_____

e-mail: _____
  (required to receive FREE health updates)

Mail in your order today!

Agora Health Books • PO Box 977 • Dept. M680HTFS • Frederick, MD 21705-9838

**For fastest service call 1-888-821-3609 and ask for code M680HTFS
or fax your credit card order to 1-410-230-1273**

PRO-I   M680HTFS